RISING

ABOVE

LYME

DISEASE

A REVOLUTIONARY, HOLISTIC APPROACH TO MANAGING AND REVERSING THE SYMPTOMS OF LYME DISEASE— AND RECLAIMING YOUR LIFE

JULIA GREENSPAN, N.D.

FAIR WINDS

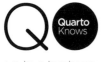

Brimming with creative inspiration, how-to projects, and useful information to enrich your everyday life, Quarto Knows is a favorite destination for those pursuing their interests and passions. Visit our site and dig deeper with our books into your area of interest: Quarto Creates, Quarto Cooks, Quarto Homes, Quarto Lives, Quarto Drives, Quarto Explores, Quarto Gifts, or Quarto Kids.

© 2019 Quarto Publishing Group USA Inc.
Text © 2019 Julia Greenspan, N.D.

First Published in 2019 by Fair Winds Press, an imprint of The Quarto Group, 100 Cummings Center, Suite 265-D, Beverly, MA 01915, USA.
T (978) 282-9590 F (978) 283-2742 QuartoKnows.com

Fair Winds Press titles are also available at discount for retail, wholesale, promotional, and bulk purchase. For details, contact the Special Sales Manager by email at specialsales@quarto.com or by mail at The Quarto Group, Attn: Special Sales Manager, 100 Cummings Center, Suite 265-D, Beverly, MA 01915, USA.

23 22 21 20 19   1 2 3 4 5

ISBN: 978-1-59233-777-4

Digital edition published in 2019

Library of Congress Cataloging-in-Publication Data available.

Cover and Page Design: Kelley Galbreath
Page Layout: *tabula rasa* graphic design

Printed in China

The information in this book is for educational purposes only. It is not intended to replace the advice of a physician or medical practitioner. Please see your health-care provider before beginning any new health program.

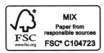

Dedicated to my mother,
Janet Geil (1948–1982),
and to my children,
Sydney and Samuel—I love you!

CONTENTS

PART 3

When Lyme Persists: It's Time to Dig Deep

INTRODUCTION

Chronic Lyme disease and associated coinfections are creating a chronic disease juggernaut that is moving through both the human body and our health care system, diminishing quality of life and productivity while increasing medical costs.

The biggest risk factor associated with Lyme disease is the denial of treatment rather than the disease itself. More than just a physical experience, Lyme disease requires a level of medical savvy patients don't even know they need until they try to find treatment for a chronic condition that many believe doesn't exist. Finding appropriate, compassionate care is a game with a unique set of rules for navigating the medical system and insurance coverage. But the stakes are high: Unresolved tick-borne disease opens the door to a range of chronic health conditions that are seemingly unrelated, including cardiovascular effects, hormone imbalance, neurological diseases, autoimmune diseases, and premature aging.

How do we rise above Lyme disease? We become educated about what to expect in the course of diagnosis and treatment, and we learn how to advocate for ourselves. My motivation in writing this book is to offer a framework for understanding the diseases ticks carry, related conditions that make recovery more difficult, the sociological impact of tick-borne disease, the trauma of trying to find help, and the range of complementary treatment options.

Rising Above Lyme Disease is a guide for patients, family members, support groups, and others, serving as a reference for treatment options, symptoms, and approaches to preventing long-term complications.

When I first considered writing the book, I pictured a chronic Lyme disease patient at home in the middle of the night, overwhelmed with fear from symptoms so intense he feels a loss of hope leading to suicidal thoughts. This scenario happens more often than most will admit. As much press as the disease gets, people with the infection still feel that they are living in the shadows, shamed for not getting well fast enough or accused of attention-seeking behavior. The more we understand the barriers a Lyme patient is up against, the more compassion we as a society will be able to give, and the more we will understand that it takes time to heal.

Tick-borne infections require patients to dig deep and learn the self-care, self-advocacy, and inner strength they will need to endure the long marathon of recovery. If they lack self-love, have experienced trauma, or have a habit of placing their needs lowest on the totem pole, they will find that these patterns hamper recovery. Life stressors, mental or emotional imbalances, and negative outlooks can be magnified during the treatment process. Neuroinflammation created by the presence of spirochetes in the brain intensifies old emotional wounds, fears, and traumas, which can dramatically slow the healing process. This is why it's so important to discuss psychospiritual aspects of the recovery process, delving into energy medicine and tapping into the innate quantum healing capabilities of the mind and body to enhance personal power, rebuild the body, and experience a deeper level of self-awareness. The healing power of the mind is substantiated by science daily, and it is a power we all have access to. Integrating conventional medical methods with alternative and energetic healing makes recovery more efficient. I have spent more than a decade weaving together multiple modalities to support patients through their journey to heal from tick-borne disease.

I am what is considered a Lyme-literate doctor with an integrative medical practice. My bachelor's degree is in psychology, and I thought I would eventually earn my doctorate in that field. Before I entered medical school, I worked as a case manager with at-risk populations in domestic violence shelters, in suicide crisis management, and in rape victim assistance. The skills I learned in my early twenties have served me well in my work with patients in crisis with tick-borne infections. Eventually, my heart felt a pull toward naturopathic medicine, and I happened to live minutes away from one of the oldest naturopathic medical schools in the country, the National University of Natural Medicine. Part of the fiftieth graduating class, I completed my doctorate in 2006 after four years of medical school, with a focus on general family practice and environmental medicine.

I had always been drawn to mind-body medicine—even in my undergraduate years—and recognized my own intuitive sensitivities in non-ordinary reality since childhood. Many people with energetic sensitivities tend to keep them quiet or dismiss them as fictional, but we all have the capacity to access our energy in a more intuitive way. We all have the capability to explain that energy away as well. To be authentic in the way I practice complementary medicine, I discuss energy healing as a way of bringing it out of the shadows. Naturopathic medicine provides a beautiful flexibility to blend science and spirit. It's an open playground for exploring all the holistic facets of medicine with a foundation of science for diagnosis and treatment. And it embraces all aspects of the human experience and honors the patient's individual journey.

The tenets of naturopathic medicine serve as my compass daily as I work with patients of all ages and from all walks of life. These tenets are:

- **First, do no harm.** This principle is about using the least invasive measures to improve a person's quality of life, working with utmost safety and integrity. Unfortunately, with Lyme disease, discomfort is often part of the healing process, but the goal is to support this process with natural medicine and lifestyle choices that minimize suffering.
- **Identify and treat the cause.** If the cause of an illness is not addressed, it will be difficult to resolve the symptoms.
- **Access the healing power of nature.** Natural medicine is not just about using herbs, nutrition, and homeopathy; it's about tapping into the innate intelligence of the body to heal when obstacles are removed.
- **View the doctor as teacher.** My role as a doctor is to empower, support, coach, and reflect compassion. Each patient is her own doctor on a daily basis, making choices for self-care. I'm the person who provides available options and gives guidance for making necessary life changes to create optimal health.
- **Treat the whole person.** Naturopathic doctors are trained to see the human body as a cooperative system instead of in parts. A doctor serves patients best when she addresses the physical, mental, emotional, genetic, environmental, social, and spiritual aspects of their lives. Treating the whole person is about listening to the complete story and understanding how to help the parts that are out of balance.
- **Support prevention.** Our job as doctors is to work ourselves out of a job by helping patients recover and avoid disease states. Prevention is the deferment of disease throughout the course of a lifetime.

I have been a Lyme-literate doctor in service to those requiring care, but I have been a patient as well. It took two years of antibiotics, herbs, homeopathy, physical medicine, and, eventually, five months of intravenous antibiotics to clear my tick-borne disease. My experience with healing modalities such as shamanism, biofield therapies, and energy anatomy is what helped me finally let go and achieve full remission. I was confirmed to have Lyme disease and was also infected with *Babesia duncani*, a tick-borne parasite. Many patients report feeling regretful and ignorant because they could not see the illness clearly enough to take action at the beginning of the infection, but try being a doctor who treats patients with tick-borne disease daily and having no idea you had it.

I explained away my symptoms for months, blaming them on the sleep deprivation that comes with having young children, a new practice, and not enough time for self-care. I could barely get myself out of bed in the mornings without feeling pain as well as vertigo. Cognition was difficult and I developed seizure-like episodes, which were very alarming for my family. It's been five years since my recovery, and I have not required treatment since. This does not mean I'm immune to being bitten again and reinfected—after all, I live in New Hampshire, among the most infested areas in the country. Throughout the process of healing from Lyme disease, I was lucky to have a medical practice centered on tick-borne infection. I had a built-in support system, with patients who offered compassionate words as I, while receiving intravenous antibiotics, met with them about their own health care needs.

With *Rising Above Lyme Disease*, I look to support you as a Lyme patient, or as a family member or friend of someone battling tick-borne illness, any way I can. I not only want to help you in resolving your disease; I want to help you realize you are not alone and we can stop the trauma cycles by becoming more informed. Be well. Take what resonates for you and leave the rest to follow your own truth.

PART

1

DEMYSTIFYING TICK-BORNE DISEASE

THE TICK: NATURE'S DIRTY NEEDLE

My naturopathic medical practice is located in southern New Hampshire, one of the most tick-infested areas of the country and one with a high rate of tick-borne disease. About halfway through writing this book, I went to work one day to find that eight follow-up patients had canceled and rescheduled. This number of reschedulings almost never happens in my office, but the coincidence brought in several very ill patients who otherwise would have waited two to three months for an appointment. When we saw the cancellations, my amazing staff got on the phone to call people on the waiting list, and within an hour we had three new patients. They represent the types of new cases we see in a typical day at the clinic.

The first patient was in her thirties, and three years earlier she'd run the Boston Marathon and worked full time in a successful career. She now suffered with chronic complaints, with her main symptoms being chronic joint pain, stabbing nerve pain, and widespread muscle pain. She reported that she had once been a very balanced person but had struggled with obsessive dark thoughts, anxiety, depression, and debilitating fatigue for the past two years. She also suffered from chronic insomnia, brain fog, sweats, rashes, hair loss, lumps under her skin, foot pain, and dizziness.

Her primary care provider (PCP) diagnosed her with anxiety and depression and prescribed medications for mood. When the patient asked her PCP to look further into tick-borne disease, the doctor refused and told her she was depressed due to her inability to have children. She asked several times to be tested for Lyme disease and other tick-borne infections but was denied because the doctor felt she was just depressed. After many visits to the doctor trying to get help with her symptoms, the patient sought a second opinion. Her lab work showed positive for Lyme disease, and we started treatment. By the next visit, approximately eight weeks later, she reported significant improvement in her mood as well as reduced pain, and she was back in the gym running again. She is still undergoing treatment for some lingering symptoms, but her quality of life has improved dramatically.

The second new patient of the day was a nineteen-year-old male who had been an Eagle Scout and straight A student up until the day, two years earlier, he woke up in the middle of the night with intense sweats and fever; he'd been suffering from overwhelming fatigue ever since. He was tested at the time and was positive for Lyme disease, but his doctor was unwilling to test coinfections. He was treated with three weeks of antibiotics at the time of initial symptoms, two years earlier. Any further treatment with antibiotics was denied.

The patient did see several specialists, including an infectious disease doctor who told him and his family that he suffered from post-Lyme syndrome and that he should go home to rest for the several months it would take to recover. No treatment was offered. So, the patient followed that advice. He did not graduate from high school, spent most of his days in bed, and was too fatigued to shower on a regular basis. He made changes to his diet, which helped the symptoms somewhat, but he was still not functional. He was unable to read for long periods of time or retain information. Though this patient has been to see many doctors and has tested positive for Lyme disease more than once, he was never given antibiotics after the initial three weeks. After being tested in my office, he was diagnosed as still having active Lyme disease and was positive for *Babesia microti*. He is recovering, after starting aggressive treatment, but because of his debilitation due to inactivity, he will have a long road to regaining his strength. Full recovery takes, on average, six months to a year, with each person's path being slightly different.

The third patient was a ten-year-old girl who'd made several visits to her pediatrician and the emergency room over a two-year span. She had several episodes of intense abdominal pain and fevers over 104°F (40°C). She also experienced chronic leg pain, headaches, and repeated sore throats with significantly enlarged tonsils. The girl's mother started to notice hair loss and mood changes in her daughter as well. She had asked to have her daughter tested for Lyme disease, but given the girl's abdominal pain, she was referred for a colonoscopy and ended up having exploratory abdominal surgery. Her appendix was removed during the surgery, even though it was not acutely infected. Though her mother had asked the pediatrician to test for Lyme in the past, she was not tested by the doctor and was never screened during any of her visits to the emergency room for a high fever. She was not tested for Lyme disease until two weeks before presenting to my clinic. Her tests were positive for Lyme disease, and we began treating her immediately.

These are three patients who were denied testing and treatment. Three patients who underwent unnecessary medical procedures or were just abandoned. Three patients who suffered because Lyme disease is not taken more seriously. Each of these patients had been to see specialists, including a neurologist, a gastroenterologist, and infectious disease specialists. I'm sorry to say that this is not an unusual occurrence for those who come to my clinic.

Lyme Disease: You Don't Get It until You Get It

You probably bought this book because you or someone you love has been diagnosed with a tick-borne disease. Arriving at an accurate diagnosis may have been a difficult journey. Perhaps you saw several doctors, chasing symptoms, and were given several diagnoses; meanwhile, you collected a binder full of lab reports and just wanted someone to listen to your story and put the pieces together. Your story might involve symptoms that come and go on a day-to-day basis, or even minute to minute. You might be fine in the morning and bedbound with pain by lunchtime. You might need people to understand that the light shines too brightly in a room or a sound is too loud, making it impossible to complete a trip to the grocery store. You may go to work every day, wondering if brain fog will cause you to make a mistake. Or you hand your young child the iPad more often than you like because you are too sick to be the active parent you envisioned.

For most people, the symptoms of tick-borne infections don't end up on the radar until the complaints are persistent and undeniable. The most poignant statement I hear is, "You don't get it until you get it." So, how do we "get" it? Learning how to advocate for yourself is important. You'll need to know how to weed through the polarized views around Lyme disease and be at peace with the process of healing. My goals with this book are twofold: to address prevention of acute Lyme disease and to focus on the physical, mental, emotional, and spiritual aspects of chronic tick-borne disease.

Chronic Lyme disease can mean big changes in daily life, affecting family structure and your ability to work. It can significantly decrease quality of life by compromising your ability to care for yourself, and it can manifest emotional trauma. Lyme disease is a unique illness that is present in broad daylight; we all know it's there and represents a problem, yet those who are sick may feel the need to hide their experiences. Most of the fear and shame patients feel, sadly, comes from their interactions with the medical profession. Healing happens when patient-doctor relationships are healthy and when patients feel supported, believed, and safe in being honest about their health concerns.

The doctor may not even be aware that a breakdown in communication is causing harm, but politics can take over, especially if the patient happens to live in an endemic area such as the Midwest and northeastern United States. The Centers for Disease Control acknowledge that Lyme disease exists, that we all need to take preventive measures to avoid tick bites, and that treatment should follow if a patient walks into a medical office with a bull's-eye rash. Far too often, however, patients are sent away having been told that the tick was not attached long enough to cause a problem or that they should wait to see whether symptoms develop. If conventional treatment is administered, it's rarely adequate, in my professional opinion. Typical treatment time for a bite or suspected bite is ten to twenty-one days of an antibiotic (and sometimes only one dose of doxycycline is given), with patients being refused treatment for longer even if they are symptomatic.

I belong to a group called the International Lyme and Associated Disease Society, affectionately referred to as ILADS. It is a collection of practitioners from around the world who believe that Lyme disease can persist and requires longer treatment time in cases where symptoms continue. Treatments are usually a combination of antibiotics to combat infection and natural medications to enhance quality of life. My practice involves both forms of treatment, and the plan is individualized based on what is best for the patient. The approach used in conventional medicine must change—and it will—but it will take time to dismantle the current belief system that chronic Lyme disease is not treatable. In the meantime, doctors who acknowledge the complexity and individual needs of healing from tick-borne disease are here to help.

One of the biggest risk factors for developing chronic tick-borne disease is a delay in treating the acute infection. Chronic Lyme disease is a complex infection that is treatable, but mainstream medicine has put forth a belief that patients must just live with "post-Lyme syndrome" with no solution.

I see the Lyme disease crisis as man-made, caused largely by the medical community's refusal to treat acute Lyme disease effectively and its denial that chronic Lyme disease exists at all. In addition, human interaction with the environment is creating widespread changes in the climate and ecology that are favorable to tick propagation. Tick-borne diseases are treatable if caught early and treated adequately—and by "adequately," I mean until the infection is resolved. Not when we say it should be resolved, but when the person has recovered in his own unique time. Specific medications and modalities may change throughout the treatment process, but it is critical to stick with a process until the infection resolves. Don't give up! The longer treatment is put off, the more difficult it is to regain optimum health.

When you discover a tick bite, take action and find a practitioner to treat it. You need to treat every tick bite as if the tick was infected. In geographic areas with high tick infestation, patients should be tested yearly for Lyme disease as part of their regular health screening. After all, if you were walking on the beach and stepped on a hypodermic needle, you would be treated with antiviral and antibacterial medications for at least thirty to sixty days to combat the worst-case scenario. A tick, attached for several hours or days, is a nature-made hypodermic needle.

Some people are cavalier about tick bites, just pulling ticks off and discarding them without a second thought. This is most common among people who have been exposed to ticks throughout their lives without perceived consequence. However, the number of infected ticks has exploded in recent decades, and we cannot count on a tick bite being harmless. Given the microbial diversity in the environment, I assume that every tick is infected. Unfortunately, many patients with new bites are turned away from medical clinics and come to see me months later, sick and angry that action was not taken sooner. They wish they had known how to better advocate for themselves.

One problem is that a large percentage of patients don't remember getting a tick bite; finding a tick on their body might have spurred them to go to the doctor right away. I have never seen a tick on my skin, but I have had two confirmed infections. If a patient is lucky enough to notice the bite and find the tick that bit him, he may not have immediate symptoms that prompt him to seek medical care. Whether tick-borne disease is acute or chronic, treating it is critical. Every day, I see patients regain a better quality of life with treatment. In some cases, the road can be long and bumpy, but it's important to be open to all treatment options, be patient with the process, and be willing to make changes in your life that align with healing mind, body, and soul.

The Life and Times of a Tick

When I give lectures describing what happens when a tick bites a human, people start to itch and squirm. It is not pleasant thinking about insects on your body, but if it makes you feel better, ticks are not considered insects. They are arachnids, in the same family as spiders, though more closely related to mites.

Growing up in Portland, Oregon, I didn't have much exposure to bugs. There were some spiders, potato bugs, worms, and the hugest slugs you can imagine. Compared with New Hampshire, Oregon was a cakewalk. I was the typical city girl who was schooled quickly when I moved to the New England countryside, with its ticks, mosquitos, black flies, fire ants, and the green horseflies that literally take a chunk out of your skin. When I first moved to the Northeast, I was even scared of dragonflies, though now they are one of my favorites.

Although people know ticks carry Lyme disease, they typically don't know ticks can also transmit other diseases. And most don't know much about the life of a tick. Understanding the life cycle and tendencies of ticks can help you protect yourself. Ticks live all over the world, with different species having evolved to survive in their particular environment. The most common tick-transmitted infections in the United States are from *Ixodes scapularis*, also known as the *black-legged tick* or the *deer tick*. It lives one to two years and has three physical stages of maturation: larval stage (newly hatched); nymph stage, which is the tick's adolescence period; and adult stage. Ticks rely on blood meals to grow into a new stage of development.

Ticks have been feeding from hosts for more than 300 million years.[1] The species vary depending on location, with *Ixodes scapularis* most commonly found in the northeastern and north-central areas of the United States and up into Canada; *Ixodes pacificus* is typically found on the West Coast in the United States as well in British Columbia; *Ixodes ricinus* occurs in Europe; *Ixodes persulcatus* is found in Europe and Asia[2]; and other species of *Ixodes* are found throughout Asia.

Ixodes scapularis is referred to as a hard-bodied tick because of the presence of a hardened cuticle that covers the entire body of a male tick and one-third of the body of a female, giving it the common two-toned elliptical shape on the back. Female ticks, larvae, and nymphs have the ability to grow tenfold in size, in both length and width, with each feeding. The male tick stays fairly small as it feeds because of its denser outer covering.[3] One of the most interesting facts about *Ixodes* is the minimal time the tick spends feeding in its lifetime. Only two to three weeks of a tick's typically 108-week life is spent actively feeding.[4] Compared with other parasites, ticks spend little time attached to their hosts, feeding only during yearly growth phases and the active reproduction phase in the female.

Newly hatched ticks are barely visible to the naked eye; they have a shape similar to that of an adult tick, with two fewer legs. These are usually free of infection but acquire infections from feeding on small rodents. However, the newly discovered strain of the bacteria *Borrelia miyamotoi* can be passed from a female tick directly to her larvae, in a process known as *vertical transmission*. This is the first time vertical transmission has been seen with tick-borne pathogens; this type of transmission will make controlling infection rates within the tick population more difficult, and the infection is likely to spread more aggressively among the population. Tests available from IGeneX and other specialty labs can now identify this strain.

The nymph stage is the most difficult to identify because the ticks are small enough that they are indistinguishable from specks of dirt. You wouldn't feel them walking on you and brush them off, and this stealth means they are also the most dangerous. They are the reason most people have no idea they have been bitten. An adult tick can be the size of a poppy seed. The strain of Lyme or other tick-borne disease a tick carries will depend on the species of tick and its geographic location. Certain strains of *Borrelia* (the genus of bacteria that includes the species that causes Lyme disease) are more apt to present with neuromuscular symptoms, while others are more likely to have relapsing fever as a symptom.

Ticks exemplify patience. They will wait months or years to feed. Their primary method of detecting a host is their sense of smell, which is far beyond that of the keenest bloodhound. This heightened sense of smell is critical because they do not have strong vision or hearing. They can detect carbon dioxide and lactic acid emissions from a host and can smell odors from microbial colonies on a person's skin. This may be the reason that certain people seem to be tick magnets, getting bitten more often than others.

Ticks do not move quickly but have amazing reflexes that allow them to grab on to a host as it walks by. Once a tick has found a host, it searches for an ideal place to feed. Because they are not fond of light, they will usually pick a place on the human body that's covered, such as the hairline, under clothing, or in areas better left to the imagination. Trust me, ticks can (and do) attach anywhere you can imagine. To feed, they use their legs and mouths to anchor themselves onto the skin. They project a jagged, razorlike appendage, making a slice in the skin where they insert their mouths to make contact with small blood vessels. Then the meal begins.

More than half of my patients with a confirmed tick-borne infection have no memory of a bite. This is because ticks prefer locations in areas not readily seen. They also release anti-inflammatory and analgesic substances in their saliva, which allows them to remain attached unnoticed. Ticks' survival depends on their ability to avoid being noticed and maintain hydration when they are not feeding. This is why areas with higher humidity and rainfall are more apt to have larger tick populations. Ticks are not sun worshippers; they prefer warm, overcast, humid days, hanging out on a blade of grass "questing" for their next meal. They maintain proper fluid balance in a variety of ways, absorbing moisture from the environment, retaining water via their waxy coating, and tightly closing body openings to reduce water release.

The tick's need to maintain moisture is also important in the transmission of disease. Over the course of hours or days, the rates of ingestion of a blood meal will vary; sometimes they feed faster and other times more slowly. Ticks need a way to manage the flow of fluid. While feeding, their salivary glands release excess fluids by regurgitating blood meal and midgut microbial content into the host, which is when infections are transmitted. The tick's midgut has a low enzyme content, which allows microbes to live there without being degraded, as food would be in the human stomach.

Ticks have a well-equipped immune system, which gives them the ability to kill invading microbes. A lot of the same processes are used by humans; however, certain pathogens have evolved to evade ticks' immune systems as well as humans'.[5] Tick saliva has many proteins that are currently being studied and analyzed for their role in the transmission of infection. These proteins reduce inflammation and pain at the bite site and also contain anticoagulants that prevent clotting of the blood in the host, enabling the tick to maintain a continuous flow of blood meal. The saliva proteins reduce immune mechanisms in the host that would ordinarily promote wound healing and attract cells to the area that would bring the host's attention to the site.[6] If this happened, the tick would most likely be removed by the host. These mechanisms have all evolved over time to enable the tick to stay attached, using its own internal medications in the form of anti-inflammatories and anticoagulants to maintain connection long enough to eat. Meals are few and far between, so ticks need to make the most of the time they are attached to a host.

Tick Attachment Time

Tick attachment time is a hot topic, and this is where politics are involved. There is much debate about how long it takes a tick to transmit infection. Many doctors tell patients that if a tick was not attached for at least twenty-four to forty-eight hours, they can throw the tick away because there is nothing to worry about. I never understood this logic. The longer a tick is embedded, the greater the risk; but ticks can transmit disease in even a short period of time. Research has shown that Powassan virus can be transmitted within fifteen minutes of a bite, while anaplasmosis and *Borrelia miyamotoi* can be passed within twenty-four hours of attachment time.[7]

The other issue is that a partially fed tick may be disturbed and drop off one host and then reattach to a new host almost immediately, posing a greater threat of infection in a short period of time. This is because, as a tick feeds, it upregulates migration of spirochetes into its salivary glands, making them transmissible. If a tick feeds on an animal or human but is removed before finishing its meal, it may quickly reattach to another host to continue the blood meal. It is then able to transmit infection soon after attaching because the spirochetes have already worked their way to the tick's salivary glands. Due to the many unknowns of the tick feeding process, the safest choice is to assume infection was transmitted, even if the attachment time was brief.

The longer a tick is embedded, the greater the risk; but ticks can transmit disease in even a short period of time.

Few people would witness the exact moment a tick implanted and think, "I've got a day or two until this becomes a problem, so let's leave it." When a tick is found, a person usually does not know the specific moment it attached—he makes an estimate. Tick attachment time is not the most reliable criterion for determining infection because the skin is numbed by the tick at the time of the blood meal, and the person doesn't feel the bite.

There are also many variables that increase the chance of infection during attachment, such as friction or pressure applied to the tick unknowingly by clothing or body movements. This can agitate the tick, which increases blood regurgitation into the host, transmitting infection. There are also other differences that come into play: the particular infections an individual tick carries, the protein makeup of that tick's saliva, the blood vessels it is able to tap into (which affects proximity of infection), and the host's immune system and skin thickness. Taking all of these variables into consideration, it does not make sense to assume the patient is in the clear.

You need to advocate for yourself to get a bite treated as soon possible. Also understand that, just because you do not see a bull's-eye rash—a red ring around the lesion—it does not mean you are not infected. A number of factors go into determining the disease process, and many who are infected do not get a rash, or indeed any symptoms, at the time of the bite. Instead, over weeks or months, their health slowly deteriorates, with confusing symptoms that seem unrelated to a tick bite. This leads to many appointments with specialists, invasive testing, and treatments that are not appropriate for the actual cause of the symptoms.

Ticks and the Environment

An ideal tick environment is shady and moist and is also home to small animals on which the tick's young can easily feed. The white-footed mouse is the primary source of infection for the larval tick because, being low to the ground, it's easy to attach to. These mice like to live in wood piles, leaf litter, and crevices of buildings, just as ticks do. The overall population of rodents, including chipmunks, squirrels, and voles, is increasing due to the warming climate and a decrease in birds of prey that would normally reduce rodent populations. Loss of habitat and viral infections have led to a significant drop in birds of prey over the past decade. Birds play a major role in transporting ticks across vast areas of the country, making it possible to encounter ticks even in New York City's Central Park or other cityscapes. With the aid of birds, ticks become mobile—like humans on a plane ride.

Trees play an important role as well by providing a food supply that lets small rodents (which transmit infection to the tick) survive a harsh winter. An increase in acorn production from oak and beech trees, called a *mast year*, seems to be happening more often in recent years. Several theories to explain mast years exist. The most plausible is that the trees' reproductive cycles take a lot of energy, so they save that energy for a larger release periodically, to ensure the tree's survival. Depending on the year, weather patterns are a driving force for bumper crops. The year after a mast year correlates to a boom in the tick population. In a study reported in *Natural Areas Journal*, researchers found that six oak trees and one hickory in Long Island, New York, experienced a mast year for three out of five years between 2007 and 2011.[8] It's not typical to have so many, but changing weather patterns in recent years have led to many events that weren't experienced ten to twenty years ago.

Although the white-footed mouse has been getting more attention because it is a well-known carrier of *Borrelia* species, most people associate Lyme disease and ticks with the deer that free-range in their backyards. Deer can carry thousands of ticks, usually adults or those in the nymph stage. Many areas are overpopulated with deer because of an imbalance of predator and prey and because of human sprawl in their migration paths. Deer and other wild animals do not want to be in our backyards, but with human development proliferating, they are running out of places to go.

There is also a big problem with moose dying off, being unable to reproduce, and collapsing because of blood loss from too many tick attachments. The warmer climate and increased tick activity have caused moose to experience thousands of tick attachments, which are creating anemia in the moose cows (females). Historically, these animals follow cold weather, moving northward in summer, and are not in infested areas at peak tick feeding time. Because of climate change, the areas they commonly migrate to have increased in temperature, allowing ticks and rodents to survive more readily.

Deer rub against trees to scrape ticks off, but moose have not yet learned this behavior. Severe blood loss is reducing the ability of moose cows to become pregnant and to deliver and feed healthy calves. In 2014, New

Hampshire Fish and Game launched a study of moose populations in New Hampshire, Vermont, and Maine to determine the impact of changing weather patterns, along with the impact of tick attachment, on the ability of moose cows to deliver healthy calves.[9] Tracking collars were placed on animals and blood samples collected to assess the health of the moose population. While numbers are reduced, the population has not yet reached the brink of destruction. It will take several years of data collection to understand the relationship between changing weather, ticks, and moose calf production.

Ticks Have No Downtime

Tick bite season is spring and fall. During these seasons, my office typically receives five calls per day about new bites. Fitting patients in right away is very important to me because the initial bite is such a sensitive time for addressing the infection. At peak season, my staff have the joy of seeing baggies and containers of ticks hanging out at the front desk more than they would care to. I have been specializing in Lyme disease for more than a decade, and over the past five or six years, tick bite calls have been growing steadily. The seasons are becoming more variable, with warmer temperatures giving the ticks more time to feed.

In 2015, in New Hampshire, we were gifted with a 70°F (21°C) day on Christmas, which was fun and weird at the same time. The following business day, we received calls for tick bites, an odd thing to treat in December. Ticks can withstand intense temperature variations and often survive best when there is a good snow pack to provide them with insulation. Deer ticks are still actively feeding in freezing temperatures, though other species may go dormant or burrow underground in the winter months. Ticks are more aggressive upon waking up in spring and getting ready to go dormant for winter, but a bite can happen any time of year.

Protecting Yourself from Ticks

You can make changes in your own environment to reduce your tick exposure. The most important step you can take is to modify the landscape of your yard: remove leaf litter; move recreational equipment such as swing sets out of shaded areas; thin excess brush to allow more light in; keep wood piles away from the house; reduce deer-attracting shrubs on the property; and monitor pests, such as mice, within the house. Clearing excess brush and leaf litter gets rid of the ideal nesting and breeding ground for rodents, reducing tick nests, too. Ideally, shrink nesting ground for mice, squirrels, chipmunks, and voles.

Placing bird feeders away from the house prevents ticks from dropping off birds into your yard and keeps at a distance the rodents who love to find ways to get into the feeders. For natural tick control in your yard, consider keeping chickens or guinea hens; these birds are ideal because they will devour several hundred ticks in a day. Chickens can clear ticks from around the house, while guinea hens prefer to spend their time in forested areas and will range in more tick-infested areas.

Another way to prevent tick bites is to use permethrin, an insecticide similar to a compound found in chrysanthemums. A neurotoxin for insects, it can be dangerous if used on human skin for prolonged periods. In minimal exposure, permethrin is reported to be nontoxic. Typically used topically for short courses of treatment for lice or scabies, it's commonly marketed under the brand name Nix. The best option for tick-bite prevention is to send personal clothing for treatment to a company such as Insect Shield or to purchase permethrin and apply it to clothing that will be used only outdoors when you need protection. This product is not meant for direct contact with the skin. Companies such as Insect Shield guarantee effectiveness up to seventy washes, so treating two to four outfits will get you through a typical spring to winter season.

While I was speaking at an event for the Holistic Mom's Network, a fellow panelist noted that she started educating her children early about ticks and the importance of changing into "special" clothes when they wanted to play outdoors. She told them they could get as dirty as they wanted but they needed to take the clothes off as soon as they were finished playing to have a bath or a tick check. She left separate totes by the door for each family member's treated clothing. Such clothing should be marked, kept separate, and washed separately. Having specially treated outfits has been important for my patients who work at jobs that expose them to ticks daily, such as in landscaping, forestry, or surveying, and for those who work in the elements to maintain public utilities.

Most people prefer to have their garments professionally treated at a modest cost rather than handling the chemicals themselves. There is much concern about using chemicals topically, especially with children because of their relatively low body weight. I typically recommend using permethrin-treated clothing or spraying commercial topical insecticides on clothes and applying more natural substances to the skin. I make that same recommendation for both adults and kids—we are never too old to take precautions as if we were newborns.

Consumer Reports performed rigorous studies with uninfected ticks and mosquitos to see how effectively each brand of the topical sprays available in the marketplace repelled ticks. The three most effective options were DEET at concentrations of 15–30 percent; Picardin by Sawyer at a concentration of 20 percent; and Lemon Eucalyptus Insect Repellent Spray by Repel at 30 percent concentration. The first two are chemical-based products, and the third is marketed as an essential oil compound. Note that the concentration of the active ingredient is important: The study found that if it went below the threshold indicated, potency was dramatically reduced, but if it was too high, the product posed toxicity risks.

Applying topical sprays, wearing treated clothing in light colors, tucking pant legs into socks, and wearing hats (with longer hair pulled up under the hat) can help you repel ticks or notice them so you can remove them before they attach. A tick is not an aggressive creature in that it is not fast moving. It is harmless until it attaches to your skin. The most effective preventions are protecting your body as mentioned above and performing regular tick checks—a meticulous inspection of the body, including the scalp, for ticks. You can also use a lint roller on you or your pets to remove ticks. If possible, shower and wash clothes immediately after coming home from potential exposure. Stay away from poorly manicured paths and tall-grass areas, especially near water.

Tick tubes are another popular method used by my patients because they minimize the need to spray chemicals in the yard. You can make these easily by spraying permethrin on cotton balls and placing them into old toilet paper rolls. The idea is that mice take the cotton to their nest, which kills any ticks before they attach to the mice. Based on a data search, this method was tested by comparing the tick count in an area treated with tick tubes and an area without. Unfortunately, there was not much of a distinction in tick population in the treated group compared with the untreated group over a two- to three-year period.[10] Note that permethrin is not selective in the bugs it kills; it will also kill pollinators such as bumblebees that make their nests low to the ground.

Sprays to treat your yard and lawn are helpful in reducing the chances you will pick up ticks. I promote the organic options for reduced toxicity to plants, pollinators, humans, pets, and wildlife. The organic formulations use synergistic combinations of essential oils (peppermint, rosemary, and geranium) together with low amounts of natural pyrethrums found in chrysanthemums as a more close-to-natural option than straight permethrin. You still run the risk of hurting pollinators, but you have the best chance of minimizing that risk with an organic spray. I am a beekeeper, so I am keyed into this issue on my one acre of land. Check your local listings for pest services that are attentive to managing pests while reducing the impact on other species of insects and on animals and humans.

There is also a garlic spray called Mosquito Barrier, which you can purchase online or in retail stores. The odor of the garlic is supposed to deter mosquitos and ticks. This method requires repeated treatment throughout the summer because the odor dissipates over time. I have seen better results and fewer treatments required when organic formulations consisting of essential oils and plant-based compounds of pyrethrum are applied by local pest control companies.

As you work to reduce your exposure to ticks, you need to consider how you will control ticks on your pets. Dogs and cats are big risk factors in humans acquiring tick-borne pathogens. I love animals and have been a pet parent all my life, but living in an area where ticks are so prevalent has changed my comfort level with having a pet. Most of my patients have an animal that goes inside and out. Cats allowed outdoors tend to pose greater risks because they venture into the brush and travel farther from home than dogs. However, cats are more easily trained to remain inside because they can use a litter box. They may not like it at first, but indoor confinement for your cats could make the difference in whether you and your family get sick. Cats that go outside may also present greater tick control challenges because they typically do not undergo tick checks willingly.

Patients have been swearing by the Seresto collar for their dogs. These flea- and tick-repellent collars have an eight-month protection period. Dog owners report few to no ticks compared with previous years. Tick repellents for cats are not easy to find because of the need to balance effectiveness and safety—the product must keep ticks away yet be nontoxic to the cat, which is difficult because of their smaller size.

Stay Calm and Tweeze On

Most of my patients don't remember being bitten, nor do they have significant evidence of symptoms immediately. If you find the tick that bit you, you're lucky, because you can take action. A wait-and-see approach is risky given the number of infected ticks in the environment. In my practice, every tick is considered infected unless its test returns clean. In many debilitating cases of chronic Lyme disease, it's not just one bite that caused infirmity. Even though the patient may remember only one bite, other ticks could have attached without the person being aware of it. Over the course of time, with each new bite, the body burden of infection grows; eventually, the infection gets to a tipping point and the body starts to show significant symptoms.

If you find a tick embedded, stay calm and resist the temptation to destroy the tick out of panic. Take a moment and gather the necessary tools: tweezers or another removal instrument such as a tick scoop; a resealable plastic bag; topical antibiotic ointment; and an adhesive bandage. Then follow these steps:

- **Remove the tick.** The best tool is a pair of tweezers or tick scoop. Some tweezers even have an attached magnifying glass that helps you see more closely. A tick scoop—a small spoon with a slice in it—acts like a hammer removing a nail. Using whichever tool you have (even if all you have is your fingers), carefully yet assertively remove the tick. Grip the tick as close to the skin as possible and try to remove it with one pull rather than repeated tugs. If the head and mouth parts are left in the skin, do the best you can to remove them. This might not be feasible without causing more trauma to the skin, in which case you can visit a doctor to have it removed.

    In most cases, the tick will naturally come to the surface of the skin to be released. Follow up with a topical antibacterial ointment on the site of the bite. The most important thing to remember is to not stress the tick with irritating substances such as garlic, kerosene, essential oils, repeated pulling, or pressing a blown-out match to its body. This will just agitate the tick to the point that it might transmit more infection by regurgitating the microbes in its gut into the bloodstream. Keep a kit for removing ticks in the house. You can purchase assembled kits that have the tweezers, container, and wound care included (the one I commonly use in my office can be purchased from Mainely Ticks). These kits usually come in small packs you can keep in the medicine cabinet or in a backpack.

- **Save it.** After you remove the tick, ideally alive or in one piece, save it in a plastic container or a small plastic bag. You do not need to add anything to the bag. Do not place the tick in alcohol, or the bacteria may not be testable. Alcohol kills or denatures proteins. If you have the tick removed at the doctor's office, specify beforehand that you want to keep the sample for testing. Otherwise, the practitioner who removes the tick might toss it in the garbage right after removal. It used to be more common practice to save the tick and have it tested, but currently many medical clinics don't seem to advocate for this.

- **Test it.** There are a lot of data in the tick, which provide clues to what might have been transmitted and help dictate the most effective treatment. Turnaround time for test results of a tick is three to five days, while it can take ten to fourteen days for your blood to show signs of infection with the tests currently available. You can send the tick to a lab and have testing done rapidly and affordably. For instance, in the New England area, TickReport (www.tickreport. com) offers testing through the University of Massachusetts. (Check with your state; some offer free or reduced-cost programs for testing.) You can also use a private lab, if you prefer.

Depending on the facility that performs the test, there are different panels to choose from, ranging in price and the number of infections tested. The most common panel screens for strains of *Borrelia*, *Babesia*, ehrlichiosis, anaplasmosis, *Rickettsia*, and tularemia (I discuss testing further in chapter 4). Depending on how many bites you get in a given season, it may or may not be feasible to test every tick. I have had ticks attached to family members tested and found the testing helpful—the labs offer real-time email updates as the tests for each infection are completed.

- **Treat it.** This step gets tricky because there are strict regulations about what constitutes a treatable case in most hospital systems. Guidelines are restrictive. If the tick test is positive for an infection, I would advise you not to take the result lightly. Many doctors prefer a wait-and-see approach; however, I would recommend treatment that lasts at least four to six weeks to avoid being on antibiotics long term in the future. You may think four to six weeks *is* long term, but this is nothing compared with the treatment time for infections that have had time to get more integrated into the body.

In my office, antibiotics paired with probiotics are the standard of care. I also commonly provide homeopathic remedies to support the system in clearing the infections. If you are not comfortable with the use of pharmaceutical antibiotics, I discuss herbal protocols with intensive dosing schedules and homeopathic nosode therapy in chapter 8. When it comes to a new bite, antibiotics blended with natural medications are the most effective way to avoid future stress. You will recover from taking antibiotics if you also take the proper probiotics to protect your gut microflora and other natural medications to support your immune system.

In Summary

Ticks are not going anywhere anytime soon. The better we understand the behavior of these little arachnids, their interaction with the environment, and the importance of protecting ourselves from bites, the better we will be at reducing transmission of tick-borne infections. Taking proper precautions by wearing permethrin-treated clothing while playing outdoors or hiking in endemic areas and using tick repellent on ourselves and our pets will significantly reduce the chances of being infected or affected long term by tick-borne infections. Even if you take all proper precautions, you may still suffer a bite.

In that case, immediate treatment can make all the difference in the path your health takes. Remember, ticks are only a problem when their bite penetrates the skin; other than this, they are harmless.

In the next chapters, we will take a more in-depth look at the bacterium that causes Lyme disease as well as other common infections carried by ticks. I will talk about other infections carried in the body that make recovery from tick-borne disease more difficult, and I'll discuss natural treatments and common antibiotics used to combat this complex illness. The more we understand, the more we are prepared to take action and receive proper treatment.

Antibiotics Vilified

I WENT INTO NATUROPATHIC MEDICINE to help people avoid taking medications, but I was raised around pharmacies and spent "Take Your Daughter to Work" days with my dad, sitting on a stool as he dispensed medications. Eventually, I worked as a pharmacy technician through college. Shortly after graduating from medical school in 2006, I moved from Oregon to New Hampshire to start a medical practice focused on environmental medicine and general family practice.

Soon, however, patients started to show up debilitated with Lyme disease. Early in my practice, I did not want to be involved in prescribing antibiotics, so I referred patients to a primary care provider for treatment. Patients would promptly return to my office, saying their doctor refused to write a prescription because they could not possibly have Lyme disease. So, I grudgingly started to write prescriptions for antibiotics. I saw people improve with a blend of natural medications and antibiotics. We doctors have a saying: "Your medical specialty picks you." Clearly, providing care in a Lyme-endemic area with a doctor shortage is mine.

Antibiotic use is a hot topic, and antibiotics once prescribed like candy are now vilified. Somewhere in the middle is the right approach for medical management of tick-borne infections. Antibiotics are not ideal solutions, but when used judiciously, they can make a positive difference. It's common for patients to feel trepidation about using antibiotics due to the drugs' impact on the gastrointestinal tract, the patients' medication sensitivity, and a general desire to take as natural a course as possible. I always respect the patient's choice, and natural medications may be exactly the right answer.

More often than not, I have seen patients improve their quality of life with the use of antibiotics, natural medications, and other healing modalities as they recover from Lyme disease. Try to stay moderate in your view, trust that recovery takes a while, and ingest those probiotics to reduce the digestive distress and secondary gut infections associated with antibiotic use. (I discuss probiotics in greater detail in chapter 7.)

CHAPTER 2

DIVING DEEPER INTO CHRONIC LYME DISEASE

L yme disease receives a lot of attention in the media and not enough during a typical doctor's visit. The disease was named after the town of Lyme, in Connecticut, where in the 1970s several children developed joint pain, fevers, rashes, and other symptoms thought to be a viral infection. In 1977, before the microbe was identified, Allen Steere, M.D., identified Lyme disease as a vector-borne illness transmitted by ticks. Most common diseases are transmitted through the air or via contaminated food or water. Vector-borne illness requires a carrier such as a tick, flea, or mosquito. A vector is an intermediary that passes infections—when ticks are the vector, infection is transmitted to the next animal during a blood meal.

In 1982, Wilhelm "Willy" Burgdorfer, Ph.D., a medical entomologist, identified the spirochete (a spiral-shaped microbe) responsible for the Lyme infection. The spirochete then was named after him: *Borrelia burgdorferi*. According to the International Lyme and Associated Disease Society (ILADS), there are five subspecies of *B. burgdorferi*, with more than one hundred strains in the United States and more than three hundred strains worldwide. Typical testing to confirm Lyme disease looks only at one strain, with specialty laboratories looking at two to four strains. This means that testing is limited in its ability to absolutely rule out Lyme disease.

Lyme Disease Is Not a New Epidemic

For a 2017 study published in *Nature Ecology and Evolution* titled "Genomic Insights into the Ancient Spread of Lyme Disease across North America," researchers did genomic sequencing on 146 genomes of *B. burgdorferi* and found that its most recent ancestor is more than sixty thousand years old. The strains active now were present at least twenty thousand years ago in North America. Remember this the next time someone tells you Lyme disease was not around before the 1970s.

According to the researchers' hypothesis, the reemergence of infection started approximately seven hundred years ago with colonization, deforestation, hunting, increased deer population, and climate change. They found no co-evolutionary relationship between the ticks and *B. burgdorferi*, but the population of *Ixodes scapularis* (deer ticks) should obviously be watched to track the presence of infection. It is uncommon for a host, in this case the tick, to have no mutually beneficial relationship with a microbe such as the spirochete. The tick serves only as a transport vessel for the spirochete without deriving any benefit from doing so.

Based on the movement of the infection over its twenty thousand–year history, it will continue to expand in all directions beyond North America.[1] The researchers' conclusion about the increase in Lyme disease over several centuries makes sense given the change in climate patterns over the past several decades, which coincides with the explosion of infected ticks. Lyme disease is present in the United States, Canada, Europe, Asia, and Australia. The most infected and infested areas of the United States are the New England area, New York, New Jersey, Pennsylvania, Maryland, Delaware, Wisconsin, and Midwestern areas, specifically Minnesota and Michigan.[2] There are also growing numbers of infections in Oregon, California, and Southern states, where many believe Lyme disease is not present. This myth makes it even harder for patients to receive treatment in states where the medical community believes there are no infected ticks and thus little to no risk of Lyme disease. TickReport has an ongoing Tick-borne Diseases Passive Surveillance database that shows reports of the diseases found in ticks tested from forty states in the United States and Canada. The number of ticks tested is always changing, but the most prevalent infections by percentage are Lyme disease (both arthritis and relapsing fever types), anaplasmosis, and *Babesia microti*.[3]

Who Counts?

IT'S HARD TO DETERMINE THE NUMBER OF PEOPLE infected with tick-borne diseases because data-reporting criteria are limited. Only those who reported a tick bite within six weeks of a positive Lyme disease Western blot (an antibody test used to diagnose Lyme disease) are factored into the numbers reported to the Centers for Disease Control and Prevention. Although the bull's-eye rash is considered the cardinal symptom, very few people develop this classic indicator. Reactions on the skin can be different, depending on the immune response at the time of the bite.

Rashes can be big and have concentric rings, but they can also be small, with just a slightly darker ring around the bite. Most of the time, however, there is nothing but a pinpoint lesion where the tick punctured the skin. The bull's-eye rash around a bite, when it does occur, is created by the spirochetes migrating through the tissue, away from the entry point into the body to find a suitable location, ideally one with low oxygen, low blood flow, low temperature, and sugar proteins. The presence of the ring is dependent on the host's immune system and the migration of the spirochetes. Given the number of variables involved in developing a rash and the number of people who don't show this symptom, it is not a suitable sign by which to judge infection.

Spirochetes and Their Movement

The bacterium that causes Lyme disease belongs to the spirochete family, and, true to its name, it looks like a spiral. The spirochete's shape allows it to be very mobile. It moves with a drilling motion that allows it to travel through denser tissues such as joint capsules, organs, and the blood-brain barrier through a process called *transmigration*. Transmigration enables spirochetes to invade tissue, triggering the host's immune system. *B. burgdorferi* can prompt the immune system to be in a continuous state of inflammation, which, over time, can cause tissue damage and premature aging. The differences in presentation for each patient with Lyme disease has to do with the person's immune system, the number of spirochetes present in the body, and other individual factors, such as genetics.

The bacteria propel themselves with a wavelike motion using a tail, called a *flagellum*. This uniquely built tail is hidden within the bacterium's structure instead of lagging behind, as in the case of a sperm cell. The presence of the flagellum is significant because these bacteria rely on motility to evade the host's immune system—with their speed, spirochetes outrun the average host's immune cells. Without the flagellum, there would be no chronic Lyme disease. Only through the spirochetes' movement are they able to cause such a havoc in the body through their ability to invade. Without that microbe's tail, our immune system and medications would more readily be able to eliminate them. You can see the host's immune response after a bite in those who develop a bull's-eye rash, called *erythema migrans*.

As I mentioned in the previous chapter, the infection moves from animal to tick to human. It is a phenomenal event for a microbe to migrate from one extreme environment to another, adapting to new surroundings in different species, from tick to mammal. There are differing temperatures, pH levels, and host immunity expression between the species. *B. burgdorferi* seems to have a unique DNA sequence, with extra genes that help it adapt in these differing environments.[4] These are microbes without a country; they are thrust into new surroundings and must adapt to a different environment within a new body. If we can look past our fears and resentment of the infection, we see that they are quite amazing resilient beings.

When microbes enter the tick's stomach, they can live in the gut for a long time between tick meals. When the tick gets ready to feed from the host, specific proteins enable movement from the tick midgut to the tick salivary gland—these are referred to as outer surface proteins (OSP).[5] The longer the tick is attached for meal, the more OSP is produced, which increases the number of spirochetes in the tick gut and salivary glands, increasing the likelihood of transmission.[6] Antibodies to these specific proteins are used to confirm exposure to Lyme disease—this is the basis for the Western blot test, which I discuss in greater detail in chapter 4.

Can You Become Immune to Lyme Disease?

Our adaptive immune system learns by coming into contact with infections, responding with antibodies, then retaining memory of the infection in order to clear it more efficiently the next time we encounter it. Unfortunately, the immune system does not retain a memory of Lyme disease, as it does for other infections. You can get Lyme disease repeatedly with each new tick bite.

According to a 2014 article published in *Infection and Immunity*, if a patient already treated for Lyme disease was exposed with new tick bites to an identical strain, she could have protective immunity for up to six years. This was only true if the exact strain was transmitted, however, and odds are not in our favor given the biodiversity in the environment.

In 1998, a published case study in the *Journal of Clinical Microbiology* detailed that skin biopsy culture of a bull's-eye rash in the same individual at two distinct times showed entirely different strains.[7]

The idea of reinfection with subsequent bites is usually not relayed to patients in literature about prevention. The possibility of reexposure is also not supported by insurance companies, which limit intravenous antibiotic therapy to twenty-eight days only once in a patient's lifetime. Typically, the first twenty-eight days are covered; subsequent treatments, if needed, are an out-of-pocket expense. Some states are creating laws to mandate coverage of Lyme disease no matter the treatment time, but in many states proposed legislation has been derailed by special interests in the insurance or medical industries lobbying against the measures.

Game Changers: New Strains with Atypical Presentation

A NEW STRAIN OF BACTERIA, *Borrelia mayonii*, was discovered in 2016 and named after the Mayo Clinic, where it was first identified. This strain is found primarily in ticks in Minnesota and Wisconsin, in the white-footed mouse, and in the American red squirrel.[8] *B. mayonii* can cause nausea, vomiting, and a rash with multiple rings appearing on the body at one time, not associated with multiple tick bites.[9] I have seen this rash presentation in the clinic many times, but because it's not recognized by most doctors, it is usually diagnosed as an allergic reaction and treated with steroids instead of antibiotics.

Another newly identified strain, *Borrelia miyamotoi*, is categorized as a relapsing fever infection; though this type of infection is usually transmitted by soft-bodied ticks, *B. miyamotoi* are carried by hard-bodied ticks.[10] Infection with this strain is associated with fever, joint pain, nausea, fatigue, and muscle aches. There are also mild to severe symptoms of hemorrhage, ranging from the appearance of broken blood vessels in skin to blood in the urine. *B. miyamotoi* was first discovered in Japan and has since been confirmed in the United States.

The Transformative Ability of Spirochetes

Spirochetes live in the body in four different forms, collected in a web of biofilm, a highly organized goolike substance that provides protection and nourishment for the microbes. These spirochete forms are spiral form, L-form, cyst form, and blebs. Over time, as they live in the body, the spirochetes transition from a spiral form by gradually straightening out, though they still have visible kinks, which gives them the appearance of the letter L.

Commonly, spirochetes enter the body in the more mobile spiral form in order to search out ideal environments to colonize. Once there, they morph into different forms within the biofilm matrix they create. The spirochete will then start to collapse in on itself, transitioning its outer covering from the membrane of an animal cell to that of a plant cell. This is the common phenomenon of the spirochete changing to different forms in the body: At all times, there are spirochetes within an infected person in the spiral form, cyst form, L-form, and blebs. The change from a long spiral with a malleable cell membrane to a more formed cell wall in the shape of a ball is amazing to see. This is a very dynamic microbe!

The spirochete colonies live in constant flux between these forms, each form requiring a different antimicrobial medication for treatment. The spirochetes will regrow, migrate, and build new colonies throughout the body. This is why symptoms seem to migrate in the body, as the immune system responds to activity in the different colonies with increased inflammation creating discomfort.

Blebs is a term representing remnants of spirochetes with DNA proteins that continue to trigger the immune system. Even without motility, they create inflammation by their mere presence. This is another explanation for the chronic nature of the infection, even after a long treatment time. Even if the spirochetes are eliminated with antibiotics, small fragments can remain in the body and trigger the immune system. It's difficult for the body to remove the debris when this disease migrates to places other infections do not typically go, such as deep into organs, muscles, joint capsules, and brain tissue. The reduced blood flow in certain areas of the body, such as the central nervous system (brain and spinal cord) and joint capsules, make it harder to heal.

Biofilm Defense

The longer the spirochetes live in the body, the more deeply they colonize tissue, living in any organ system. These colonies are dynamic collectives within a living matrix called *biofilm*. When seen under a microscope, biofilm is like a slime organized in elegant structures; created by several species of bacteria, biofilms control population growth of the bacteria, sequester nutrients, and provide protection against external assault.[11] It's a natural process of bacteria that predates humans. The most common biofilm, called *plaque*, is in your mouth. Scientist Antonie van Leeuwenhoek discovered biofilms in 1684, when he noticed that some bacteria were unable to survive exposure to vinegar in the mouths of animals while those bacterial cells encased in the slime matrix did survive.[12]

Made up of minerals, extracellular DNA, and polysaccharides, biofilm is able to adapt to its environment and adjust to pH, host defense, and temperature, and to make intelligent modifications based on the competition of other bacteria for nutrients. With biofilm responsible for 65 percent of all chronic infections globally,[13] it's one of the major reasons Lyme disease is so difficult to resolve. The bacteria within the biofilm would most likely be susceptible to medications, but the medications cannot penetrate the biofilm effectively enough to reduce the population of the pathogen, so it persists. This is a different process from a microbe evolving to become antibiotic resistant on its own in the environment.

Inhibiting biofilms is important when treating tick-borne disease. Bacteria have an amazing ability to create natural barriers that block incoming assault, as well as an ability to pump out invading toxins before they can cause harm.[14] As the microbes settle in, they create a biofilm that makes *B. burgdorferi* a thousand times more resistant to antimicrobial therapies. Eva Sapi, Ph.D., and others have been studying the behavior of biofilms to understand how they grow, what they are made up of, and how to improve clinical outcomes by learning what substances penetrate it.[15] Ongoing research is looking for both pharmaceutical and natural medications to dismantle biofilm and inhibit *quorum sensing*, bacteria's method of communication to maintain healthy populations in response to their environment. Herbs such as turmeric/ curcumin, garlic, oil of oregano, berberine, and green tea extract have been shown to be viable options for their anti-biofilm and anti–quorum sensing properties. Once these mechanisms are inhibited, the medications can more effectively reach the *Borrelia*.

Sometimes the terms *biofilm* and *bacterial antibiotic resistance* are used synonymously, but these are two different things. Antibiotic resistance is the ability of the bacteria themselves to be resistant to a particular treatment. This is also very different from the view held by many patients that they will become resistant. It's not the person who becomes resistant but the microbes. This is a bigger issue than one person taking medications. The biggest contributors to antibiotic resistance are the improper waste disposal of antibiotics into the waterways and massive medicating of livestock with antibiotics, which are then released in pastures onto the microbes in the soil. With biofilms present, the bugs are susceptible to medications in many cases but are protected by biofilm.

Signs of Acute Infection

A majority of my patients are chronic Lyme disease sufferers. However, each one started with an acute manifestation that could possibly have been nipped in the bud if they had been treated appropriately at the time of the bite. Treating acute cases is rewarding because I can help people avoid months or years of suffering.

The difficulties in getting treatment for acute bites are discussed throughout the book. When treatment is given, it's commonly one capsule of doxycycline, which is not enough to kill the spirochetes. One capsule of doxycycline has been proven ineffective but remains the treatment recommended by the Centers for Disease Control.[16] No other routine bacterial infections are treated with a single dose of an antibiotic, yet this is deemed adequate for a complex migrating microbe such as a spirochete. Other infections transmitted along with Lyme disease make the scenario more complicated, warranting treatment for at least thirty days with a new bite. With an acute Lyme disease infection, patients can experience symptoms within twenty-four hours to fourteen days. There may also be no major symptoms to raise concern, making it more likely to become a chronic infection.

The rash can exhibit the classic bull's-eye that is a few inches in diameter, or it can present as multiple rings. It may also be one giant ring spanning the length of the leg or across the torso. Many patients report that they initially did not seek medical care for their tick bites because no ring rash formed. Slowly, over the course of a couple of months, they started to notice they were more fatigued, with body aches, swollen joints, neck pain, headaches, vertigo, rashes, fevers, and chills.

One of the most dramatic symptoms that can accompany Lyme disease is Bell's palsy, though I have seen very few cases of acute Bell's palsy in my years of practice. This condition is caused by inflammation of the seventh

Lyme disease is consistently inconsistent.

cranial nerve, which leads to weakness and a loss of tone on one side of the face. This can impair a person's ability to speak clearly and may create visual impairment with a drooping eyelid. This symptom can resolve with treatment, returning the face to normal symmetry. People are frequently diagnosed with Bell's palsy due to viral infection, so they are not given antibiotics. When Bell's palsy continues for a long period of time, the face may not regain true symmetry; however, there can be improvement with treatment, even in later-stage cases.

When Acute Lyme Disease Becomes Chronic

Chronic Lyme disease is known as The Great Imitator. It can look like many autoimmune diseases, including rheumatoid arthritis, lupus, Sjögren's syndrome, or mixed connective tissue disease. It's also commonly misdiagnosed as a neurological disease, such as Parkinson's disease or multiple sclerosis. Arthritic and/or neurological diseases may also exist in the body along with Lyme disease and can create enough stress on the immune system to set other disease processes in motion.

Lyme disease has different stages of severity, referred to as *early disseminated infection* and *late disseminated infection*. Early disseminated infection can last weeks to months if the acute infection is not treated. Late disseminated infection can last months or years, with neurological symptoms progressing over time. Symptoms are commonly found in multiple areas of a patient's body, with complaints of musculoskeletal pain, neurological symptoms, cardiorespiratory symptoms, endocrine imbalance, skin lesions, and gastrointestinal problems. The symptoms come and go, migrating through the body with no rhyme or reason.

Spirochetes love areas of the body that have low blood flow but are high in fat and sugar, such as connective tissue, joint capsules, and nerve tissue such as the brain, which is mostly fat. These microbes can live anywhere, even landing in scar tissue because of the reduced circulation in those areas. Lyme disease is consistently inconsistent. This you can rely on. It's just plain confusing for patients and doctors who are used to the presentation of infections being more reliable. The location of the tick bite and the specific infections introduced into the system have a lot to do with this variability.

The first thing I ask patients at the beginning of a visit is when they last felt well. From there, I ask to hear the patient's story before moving to my office and reviewing their symptoms from head to toe. I see in people's eyes a look of relief because they had been thinking all this time that they were experiencing an unexplained phenomenon. They may have brought their symptoms up to doctors in the past, only to be met with responses that caused them embarrassment as they were told their feelings were irrelevant and they should seek counseling. One example of a commonly dismissed symptom, thought of as a sign of mental imbalance, is a sensation like bugs creeping on the skin. Patients are always relieved to know I saw several people in the office before them that day with the same symptom. I experienced it myself, and this was the symptom that finally got my attention and prompted me to look deeper into my own Lyme disease.

Can I Transmit Lyme Disease to My Partner?

At some point, a patient will ask me about the possibility of transferring Lyme disease to a partner through sexual relations. The topic of transmission by human-to-human contact is an important one, and there is a great deal of misinformation out there. I have counseled many patients who already feel isolated and misunderstood when they tell others they have Lyme disease, and they are now abstaining from sexual intimacy or even kissing for fear of passing the disease to another person. This is a burden people carry in addition to their diagnosis.

Transmission through saliva has not been proven; however, some Internet research and the varying opinions of medical professionals can leave a traumatizing impression. It is highly unlikely that *Borrelia* spirochetes survive in saliva given the oxygen-rich microenvironment of the mouth. Some microbes can persist either inside or outside the body; however, *B. burgdorferi* is very sensitive to its environment, and the oral cavity is not a viable place for it to thrive. If it were easy to catch Lyme disease from a kiss, it would be a global epidemic rather than one dependent on geographical areas with environments ideal for ticks.

There is a distinct possibility, however, that Lyme disease can be sexually transmitted. In a 2015 study of twelve couples, *B. burgdorferi* was cultured out of vaginal secretions and semen, and the couples had identical strains in their samples.[17] This was an important finding, prompting deeper research to understand how Lyme disease can be transmitted sexually. Gregory Bach, D.O., had observed in 2001 that monogamous couples with one partner who had confirmed Lyme disease typically had more antibiotic failure.[18] Of course, many people carrying Lyme disease do not know it and may pass it through intimate acts. It's also important to mention that most partners have similar exposure to ticks because they live on the same property and engage in many of the same activities.

When fear that Lyme disease could be spread from person to person first made its way through the Lyme disease community, I was asked about it almost daily. Many couples came in crying, and women worried they had infected their husbands. This possibility has an adverse effect emotionally and is difficult to manage on top of the other stressors within relationships when chronic Lyme disease is involved. Often, women seem to carry this burden emotionally, as if they are to blame. I've witnessed some unpleasant interactions between couples, with one partner blaming the other for giving him or her Lyme disease. Until there is more research on this topic and we understand the incidence of transmission more clearly, I encourage people to step away from the language of blame within relationships.

Based on the preliminary data, it would be wise to use barrier methods during sex while undergoing treatment for tick-borne infection, not only to protect your partner but because it could help resolve the infection more efficiently by avoiding passing it back and forth. More research is needed to understand the sexual transmission of Lyme disease. In the meantime, you should fully enjoy intimacy but take precautions.

Mother-to-Child Transmission

I have treated many women with Lyme disease and other tick-borne infections who report having a difficult time getting pregnant or having had more than one miscarriage. Pregnant patients with a history of chronic Lyme disease or who are infected during pregnancy may have positive cord blood tests in their newborns. This means transmission occurred either in utero or during the birth process. Cord blood testing involves taking a sample directly from the cord before it is cut. For the purposes of identifying the presence of infection, all tests that would commonly be run on an adult can be run on a newborn through their cord blood, where mother and child's blood intermingle through the birth process. I would recommend doing a Western blot to check for contamination of the cord blood (mother's and infant's blood commingled) as well as a culture to check for the growth of spirochetes within the infant's blood. Both would be helpful in eliminating questions about transmission; the infant's antibodies are not developed enough at the time of birth to make the information of the Western blot reliable as a primary source.

If the result is positive, Lyme disease was transmitted, and both mother and baby should be treated by a Lyme-literate doctor. I have had several pregnant patients with active Lyme disease—who either had it before they conceived or who contracted it during pregnancy—give birth to healthy children. It's important, if mom is suspected or confirmed as having Lyme disease, that she be treated.

The protocols I follow for treating during pregnancy, infancy, and up to adolescence are based on those created by Charles Ray Jones, M.D., one of the foremost experts in pediatric Lyme disease in the world. I have had the privilege of learning from him by cotreating patients and seeing him speak on several occasions. I am so grateful for his work and contributions to the Lyme community. Treating during pregnancy is delicate, and only antibiotic medications safe in pregnancy are used.

Peer-reviewed journals feature articles referencing the increased incidence of cardiac and other physical malformation in babies whose mothers have been exposed to Lyme disease.[19] However, many articles state the opposite, making it difficult to know how to proceed. There are several articles on the impact of *Babesia* species in pregnancy, with most case studies involving the treatment of the pregnant patient and screening of the newborn via blood smears. Mother and baby were reported healthy at follow-up a few months after delivery. Most of the studies of vertical transmission—transmission from mother to child instead of from a tick—have been conducted with animals such as voles and mice and show a high rate of transmission.[20]

Many mothers with positive titers (a measure of the presence and number of antibodies in the blood) for Lyme and other tick-borne diseases report having children with poor attention, difficulty learning, sensory integration issues, and increased incidence of allergies. Clinically, these are common reports on a pediatric patient's health history from their parents, who thought they just had a colicky baby. Mothers with infected children usually wonder if they gave the disease to their children during pregnancy. It's deeply painful to find out you may have infected your own child with Lyme disease.

I was infected in 2009, during my third trimester of pregnancy. At the time, I was very ill, with a high fever and intense body pain for over a week. I thought it was the H1N1 viral infection prevalent that year. After my son was born, my recovery was really difficult. I was in pain daily, could not lose the baby weight, was emotionally out of balance, felt dizzy, had night sweats, and suffered from chronic headaches and brain fog. At the time, I had a two-year-old daughter and a newborn and was getting a new clinic off the ground. I was exhausted, but it was easy to blame my symptoms on circumstances. This line of thinking delayed my treatment. Even a Lyme-literate doctor can downplay symptoms, despite her job discussing Lyme disease with patients every day.

I tell moms to put a time limit on their self-blame or grief. It's important that they be allowed to process their emotions but not to punish themselves. I see mothers carry shame and guilt for years over feeling they are the cause of their child's infection. Many manage their fear by spending every spare moment researching a cure for the child, to the point that they are not engaged in family relationships. Life becomes all about the illness. It's easy to understand the motivation behind it, but a hyperfocus on any one thing is not healthy. Even when the child starts to recover, a mom or dad may not be able to see it because the search has been a part of their lives for so long.

Age-Specific Challenges of Lyme Disease

Children have a unique experience with Lyme disease. I routinely treat infants and toddlers who have minimal verbal skills after a tick bite or positive test for Lyme disease. The most common age groups at risk for tick bites are those aged two to fifteen and thirty to fifty-five. Children ages five to ten years are especially at risk because they are low to the ground, favor play structures near the forest line or in the shade, and have thinner skin than toddlers. Depending on the age of the child and the level of awareness they have about ticks, they may also be more likely to pull a tick off without telling a parent or teacher. This is why it's important to start tick awareness with children as early as possible, so they will know to tell you if they see one on their body.

It's easy if a parent brings the child in after a Lyme disease–positive tick was pulled from the child and tested through a lab. This means we have pretty conclusive evidence of exposure. I'm not willing to take the risk of waiting to see whether there are any ill effects. Thankfully, tick testing usually encompasses not just Lyme disease but a panel of tick-borne infections. This can be really helpful in choosing the right medication from the get-go.

If your child is bitten but you never find a tick, the child may get a fever, joint pain, and a red ring around the bite site. However, he may just slowly over time have a change in personality with slight complaints of stomach pain, leg pain, and headache. Many parents, with loving intention, question whether their child is just trying to get attention until the symptoms are undeniable. They then take their child to the pediatrician, who is not comfortable testing or treating if there is no history of known tick bite. Parents know there is something wrong with their child, but most end up with a diagnosis of behavioral problems, attention deficit disorder, or an auto-immune disorder requiring intense medication regimens that are likely not needed.

As children mature into teenagers, Lyme disease symptoms can amplify due to hormone changes in both genders and the onset of menses in girls. Where there were just random complaints of headaches, stomachaches, and difficulty concentrating, there may now be debilitating fatigue and a constellation of symptoms listed above. The immune system, together with the fact that this is a time of growth and develop-ment, complicates the symptoms. Over the years, I have seen many cases of teenagers well past the time they would be expected to show signs of pubertal changes who have not begun to develop. A teen of fifteen may maintain the body of an eleven-year-old. Once the infection is identified and treated, they start maturing almost overnight.

As children mature into teenagers, Lyme disease symptoms can amplify due to hormone changes in both genders and the onset of menses in girls.

Teenagers and college kids add another layer of complexity by having an illness smack dab in the middle of teen rebellion years and at a time when so many expectations are placed on them. Many will reject their medications, make poor food choices, and resent any attempt to provide medical care. Others will continue to participate in high-impact sports and try to keep the same course load out of a fear that they will not be successful enough. This is not true of every teenager, but it does come up with many.

The most difficult situation arises when they are not able to attend school and fall behind. Some school administrations are very supportive and empa-thetic, but I have unfortunately dealt with many schools that penalized families for truancy because the school fails to accept Lyme disease as a serious illness. Even for teens who enjoy being with their families, being at home and losing social connections at this stage in their lives can be very stressful. The good news is that most kids who require homeschooling return to school and usually catch up quickly.

I treat several adolescent patients who are extremely compliant but also kids who want nothing to do with a diagnosis of Lyme disease. Many believe their parents are just paranoid. Avoiding treatment just delays recovery. Most young people who did not take treatment seriously finally decide to treat when they are over the age of twenty and they step into maturity managing their own health. Often, their resentment and rejection of treatment is rooted in fear. If they have been raised with a parent or sibling who has been ill most of their lives, it's frightening to be the one to face the disease, which can cause them to flee from the situation. Most of the time, though, kids recover from tick-borne disease more easily than adults; this is not to say it is easy, by any means—just easier.

A Symptom Profile of Chronic Lyme Disease

The symptoms presented here are those I see on a daily basis. Many Lyme disease symptoms overlap with those of coinfections, so finding the right treatment sometimes requires trial and error. Symptoms noted below are based on the most common presentations, but the list is not exhaustive.

HEAD, EYES, EARS, NOSE, AND THROAT

Most Lyme patients complain of headaches, which can be a daily occurrence. Many just get used to them. All types of headaches can manifest; typically, they are centered behind or above the eyes or radiate from the back of the neck, over the top of the head. They also vary in intensity, from a dull ache to an intense migraine that limits activity. Frequency can vary between constant daily pain or flare-ups every few weeks. The most common presentation is a constant low-level headache that gets in the way of concentration; this needs to be factored in when kids are labeled as having focus and attention issues. If a child has had Lyme disease from a young age, he may have learned to compensate and live with the pain.

Many patients also experience a sensation of being lightheaded, with or without a headache; sometimes, the lightheadedness is accompanied by more debilitating forms of vertigo such as dizziness upon standing or a continuous sensation of instability that limits daily function. This can be accompanied by brain fog or a feeling of being mentally/emotionally dissociated. The vertigo can be related to inner ear inflammation caused by the presence of spirochetes in the central nervous system, or it may be related to a cardiovascular abnormality, with blood return to the brain. Prescription medications, homeopathics taken at the time of vertigo episodes, or acupressure wristbands (brand name Sea-Band) can reduce the severity. Sea-Band is an affordable drug-free remedy and can be purchased at your local pharmacy.

Changes in vision are typical. The most common symptoms reported are light sensitivity, spontaneous blurred vision, blind spots, and abnormal phenomena, such as orbs, in the field of vision. Floaters can be dark spots, sparkles, or tracers; just about everyone with chronic Lyme disease has floaters in their field of vision. These may also look like squiggly lines. Patients report floaters that look like a spirochete itself moving across their field of vision; however, this is not actually a spirochete, since they are too small to see with the naked eye.

Over the years, I have also seen many patients become unable to drive because they get disoriented and visually overstimulated while in the car. Even riding as a passenger can present problems, and some patients require time to reorient themselves once they arrive at the clinic before the visit starts. Many patients wear blackout masks to prevent sensory overload. Several have gone months or years without being able to drive on their own.

Light sensitivity requires many patients to wear sunglasses both outdoors and indoors. I have dimmers on the lights in my office so I can adjust lighting for patient comfort. An eye exam often shows that patients have dilated pupils due to adrenal fatigue from the stress of prolonged illness, which can also create more sensitivity to light. Uveitis, inflammation of the middle layer of the eye, is common with tick-borne disease, most commonly with *Borrelia*, *Bartonella*, and *Rickettsia* species with a genetic marker of HLA-B27.[21] Many patients also have uncomfortable sensations of burning and dry eye. Most require an eye specialist as they move through treatment.

Tinnitus (ringing in the ears) is the most common change in hearing. Many different sounds are reported—such as clicking, popping, hissing, and ringing—which reduce the ability of the patient to hear. Tinnitus can be isolated in one ear or may occur in both. In most cases, it is the presence of a tone that causes varying levels of annoyance. Many patients are erroneously diagnosed with Ménière's disease, which is vertigo with tinnitus and hearing loss. Some patients experience pain or itching in the ear canal.

A handful of patients require sound-cancelling headphones to combat a debilitating symptom called *hyperacusis*, a hypersensitivity to everyday sounds. This condition can be downright painful and may require significant micromanagement of daily life to minimize the negative sensation of sound. If a patient reports hyperacusis, I always recommend counseling to help them develop coping mechanisms and support the trauma associated with phono-phobia (fear of sound) and isolation from social situations due to the discom-fort created by even soft sounds. Individuals with long-term hyperacusis develop depression and anxiety due to avoidance of sound triggers.

Retraining the nervous system response using neural biofeedback, hypnotherapy, or pink noise therapy can be a valuable way of managing stress. Like the white noise commonly used in sleep sound machines or fans, pink noise is reduced in intensity and features softer tones. Exposure to this noise can decrease the awareness of the tinnitus or expose those with hyperacusis to bearable sounds so they gradually become able to tolerate more noise.

Sinus headaches are very common, together with an increased incidence of persistent sinus infections, which may have been in the body prior to contracting Lyme disease but are more active with a weakened immune system. Nasal swab culture testing can identify the strain of infection as well as the presence of antibiotic-resistant infections in the sinus cavity. The treatment chosen is based on the susceptibility of the strain of sinus infection to certain medications.

Recurrent sore throats, with or without enlarged tonsils, are very common. This can be due to chronic strep and Epstein-Barr infections related to mononucleosis, which can become more active once Lyme disease is in the body. These are opportunistic infections that emerge in a host with a weakened immune system. They can cause enlarged lymph nodes and pain in the head and neck, as the body's immune system tries to clear the infection. Upon medical exam, most patients have enlarged tonsils and report pain as well as changes in voice quality.

NERVOUS SYSTEM

Neurological symptoms can range from subtle annoyances to debilitating experiences. They will arise depending on the location of the infection and how long it has been present in the body. Patients sometimes come to me having been diagnosed by a neurologist with amyotrophic lateral sclerosis (ALS, also known as Lou Gehrig's disease), Parkinson's disease, or multiple sclerosis. Yet over time the disease does not show the typical progression and the medications prescribed do not have the expected impact. The long-term presence of infections living in the nervous system can be a catalyst for the aforementioned diseases, and repeated cycles of inflammation caused by long-term infections can destroy neurons.

Research reported in the *Journal of Neuroinflammation* in 2013 found that Lyme disease creates inflammation markers that specifically target peripheral nerve cells and the regenerative components of the nervous system, called the *glial cells*.[22] It's an attack by your own immune system on the pathogen, but it damages tissues as a side effect. The myelin sheaths covering and protecting nerves are altered, which leads to improper transmission of information and, ultimately, pain or loss of sensation. This does not happen overnight but over the course of years, after several bites from ticks and the resulting long-running attack on tissues by the immune system.

Neurological symptoms run the gamut, representing decreased or increased activity in the neurological system. Decrease of function includes loss of motor skills, slowed processing of information, depressed mood, and loss of sensation in different areas of the body. This potentially leads to altered gait, weakness, muscle wasting, difficulty swallowing, numbness in multiple areas of the body, and/or altered speech patterns, including slowed speech, slurred speech, stuttering, and difficulty with word recall.

An overactive neurological system can create muscle twitches, tremors, increased pain, itching of the skin, burning sensations, anxiety, seizures, tics, rapid speech, and hyperactivity. Other symptoms seen in very advanced stages of infection include an inability to write clearly and even a complete change of personality. Many patients present to the clinic with their only symptom being slowed speech, or dysphonia. This is a difficult symptom to reverse, and each patient I have personally seen with this symptom has tested positive for Lyme disease.

MUSCULOSKELETAL SYSTEM

The musculoskeletal system includes joints, muscles, tendons, ligaments, fascia, and bones. Pain, swelling, weakness, increased joint instability, and reduced function due to pain are common. Symptoms may migrate throughout the day, with a patient feeling knee pain in the morning that radiates to the hips in the afternoon, moves from side to side, and ends the day in the neck. Commonly, joint swelling comes and goes with no pattern. Symptoms can be isolated in one spot, such as a knee, hip, hand, neck, spine, or foot, or may be felt in multiple places at one time.

Most patients have been diagnosed with fibromyalgia before they come to the clinic; this is a formal diagnosis of fatigue and widespread pain in the muscles. This diagnosis describes symptoms but not why the muscles hurt. The body is intelligent, having evolved to survive on this planet, and there is a reason the muscles are sore. Is it always infection? No. Does infection need to be evaluated as a cause? Yes.

Pain typically escalates with initial treatment for Lyme disease, and this is the number one reason that treatment fails. Patients often elect to stop medications because the pain is too intense; however, treatment can be modified to reduce the intensity. Most patients have been diagnosed with rheumatoid arthritis, ankylosing spondylitis, juvenile rheumatoid arthritis, Sjögren's syndrome, sarcoidosis, mixed connective tissue disease, or another condition. Patient labs can show elevated rheumatoid factor, antinuclear antibodies, sedimentation rate, and C-reactive protein in reaction to the presence of spirochetes in their tissues. More often than not, however, just one marker is elevated, with no other blood results confirming autoimmune disease.

A study published in 2017 in the journal *Arthritis and Rheumatology* showed that *B. burgdorferi*–infected joint capsules had an increase of proteins meant to initiate antibacterial action. This protein increase also happens with synovial fluid (fluid in a certain type of joint), which shows bactericidal activity in situations of septic arthritis when there is staph infection in the joint. Chronic Lyme disease increases proteins associated with chronic inflammation, which

Autonomic Dysfunction

THE AUTONOMIC NERVOUS SYSTEM (ANS), part of the peripheral nervous system, regulates blood pressure, urinary function, stress response, sweating, and digestion. The two primary areas governing function are the sympathetic and parasympathetic nervous systems. The sympathetic nervous system controls the fight-or-flight response, while the parasympathetic controls the rest-digest response.

Autonomic dysfunction, or dysautonomia, is the inability of the ANS to behave as it typically would in coping with moment-to-moment life stress to maintain balance. This commonly happens with chronic conditions such as Lyme disease, autoimmune disease, and diabetes.

Lyme disease microbes can migrate and have an affinity for nerves, which causes abnormal function. The nerves of the ANS are no exception. Patients who display autonomic dysfunction are more likely to be diagnosed as having conversion disorder or psychosomatic illness. This is because Lyme disease is very difficult to diagnose and may seem purely a manifestation of poor coping skills. Autonomic imbalance can also lead to low blood pressure, referred to as orthostatic hypotension, and postural orthostatic tachycardia, characterized by dizziness on standing. Both these conditions represent the body's inability to maintain proper heart rate and blood pressure when moving from a sitting to a standing position. The constriction or dilation of blood vessels is mediated by the autonomic nervous system, and it makes adjustments as we move, moment to moment. Fainting can be the consequence of this imbalance, and it can happen at inconvenient times in public places. Improper ANS response can also cause bladder control issues, slowed gastric emptying, sweating, poor exercise tolerance, and shortness of breath.

Many patients with these symptoms are labeled as mental instable, as the symptoms are viewed as purely anxiety driven. There is an anxiety component, certainly, as patients who have involuntary physical symptoms may be afraid to go out in public. Most require a gentle environment and micromanagement of stressors so as not to trigger fainting. Over the years, I've had several patients who have lost consciousness in my office, even with my best efforts to maintain a peaceful situation. Just getting through an office visit in which they are reporting symptoms can be too much for some.

Patients respond well to intravenous electrolyte hydration, increased electrolytes in the diet, and adrenal support. Many require conventional medications to regulate blood pressure, often taking medication to raise their pressure. Studies have shown that meditation and yoga can be helpful in improving autonomic function in patients with advanced neurological impairment.[23]

is inflammation without resolution. This causes poor wound healing or leads to tissue with reduced integrity.[24] It's especially complicated for patients with an HLA-B27 marker present because they are more likely to develop persistent autoimmune reactions that impact the eyes and musculoskeletal system. If this marker is present in a patient, it is probable that her most persisting symptoms will be joint pain and visual abnormalities.

Most of the conventional treatments for autoimmune diseases are geared toward symptom management, typically chemotherapeutic medications, steroids, and anti-inflammatories. There are times when steroids and anti-inflammatories are needed to care for severe conditions, but these drugs carry a high risk of side effects. If long-term use of steroids to manage the symptoms of an autoimmune disease is being recommended to you, I would urge you to get a second opinion from a naturopathic practitioner or someone trained in complementary medicine. If natural medicine offers no different answers, you can always return to the path of palliation with steroids, which may ultimately be the right answer for you. Most patients are nervous of taking medications, including the ones I recommend, but when push comes to shove, most patients opt to take a medication that will help resolve their symptoms.

ENDOCRINE SYSTEM

No matter the infection—whether it is bacterial, viral, parasitic, or fungal—the endocrine system is affected. The system is usually thrown out of balance, either overproducing or underproducing hormones. The endocrine system manages immune function in the body and includes glands and their cross-communication with other organ systems. The glands most commonly evaluated are ovaries/ testes, adrenals, pancreas, thymus, thyroid, parathyroid, pituitary, and pineal. The function of almost all the glands can be tested via either blood work or saliva.

In evaluating the status of the hormone system, I'm interested in body temperature, blood pressure, female hormone cycles, libido in both genders, weight status, cravings, and energy level. Typically, patients present with low body temperature, in the range of 97.7°F (36.5°C) or below. This most commonly happens because of low thyroid function. Many patients have a low-functioning thyroid and require hormone replacement. Common complaints with low-functioning thyroid (hypothyroidism) are an inability to lose weight, low libido, debilitating fatigue, dry skin, sluggish bowels, sugar/salt craving, and low blood pressure. Hypertension can also be an issue with hypothyroidism.

A majority of my patient population are women ages twenty to sixty years. This is consistent with the average patient population in a given general practitioner's office, as women seem to be more open to seeking medical attention and more in tune with changes in their bodies, especially

Insult to Injury

LYME DISEASE SYMPTOMS COMMONLY EMERGE after a trauma to the body in the form of physical injury or a major life stressor. Old injuries can start to act up again when a patient has Lyme disease. For example, a patient who had surgical repair to a knee or shoulder years earlier may begin to experience pain and stiffness again. Spirochetes have a habit of colonizing in scar tissue because these areas tend to be cooler and more prone to inflammation, having a weaker tissue matrix due to previous injury and reduced blood flow. There have been many cases over the years—with injuries as simple as a collision on the soccer field or as serious as a car accident—where the person does not recover in a typical time frame because of dormant Lyme disease. The patient might develop migrating joint pain, headaches, fatigue, and neurological symptoms, though there were none before the injury.

If you have an injury that is not healing in a proper time frame, consider that infection may be the cause. If you live in an area endemic for Lyme disease or have visited one on vacation, you may have been exposed to tick-borne infection even if you don't remember a bite. For the most accurate result, ask to have a Lyme Western blot test run (see chapter 4 for more on testing). Speak with a Lyme-literate medical professional to ensure that you are treated properly and in a timely way.

irregularities in their periods. Women with chronic Lyme disease almost always have changes in menstruation, including periods that are too heavy, too light, too short, too long, absent, or accompanied by intense pain. They may also experience early menopause, infertility, repeated miscarriages, and an intensification of tick-borne symptoms before their periods. The beauty of this sign of imbalance is that normal function usually resumes as they recover, indicating a return to health.

Many women have estrogen dominance with low progesterone due to prolonged stress and genetic predisposition. Estrogen makes tissue grow, and progesterone helps tissue develop properly, particularly in the lining of the uterus. A hormone imbalance with estrogen dominance leads to endometriosis, fibroid development, and other cycle irregularities, such as periods that are too heavy and too lengthy. Cycles that in healthy adult females average twenty-eight to forty days occur every fourteen to twenty-one days in Lyme patients. This leads to excessive blood loss, causing iron deficiency and fatigue. Such irregularities are usually caused by altered communication between the brain and the uterus as well as between the adrenals and ovaries. This miscommunication is due to the long-term stress on the system that chronic Lyme disease causes.

Men may experience low libido and low testosterone levels at younger ages than would normally be seen. Just as women pass through menopause, men go through andropause, a natural, age-related decrease of testosterone. However, I am seeing men in their twenties who have hormone levels like those of men in their seventies. Men can also become overly estrogenic as part of the stress on their bodies. Low testosterone in both genders can lead to reduced muscle mass, low energy, poor wound healing, and premature aging.

Debilitating fatigue is the most common hormone-related symptom of Lyme disease, other than pain.

Debilitating fatigue is the most common hormone-related symptom of Lyme disease, other than pain. Fatigue creates a vicious cycle of stress because patients want to maintain their usual pace of life. This leads to anxiety and depression as they worry about not measuring up. High levels of fatigue can affect a person's ability to be an active parent, maintain a job, and care for a home and relationships. Most fear not being the person they were before they got sick and becoming a burden to their loved ones. Debilitating fatigue is typically due to adrenal fatigue; in this condition, the glands sitting atop the kidneys are depleted by prolonged stress, disrupting the hormones that support proper sleep cycles, insulin sensitivity, energy levels, and cellular repair. For all my patients, I advise supporting the adrenals with herbal compounds as a standard of care. Adrenal glands can be tested for their level of function, which I will discuss in chapter 4. Typical symptoms of adrenal fatigue are energy decline after lunch together with sugar cravings, caffeine use, weight gain around the middle, and sleep disruption.

SKIN, HAIR, AND NAILS

Skin can show signs of poor wound healing, stretch marks, brittle nails, fungal overgrowth on skin/nailbeds, hives, tinea versicolor (a fungal infection of the skin), easy bruising, fast-growing spider veins, Raynaud's syndrome, creeping sensations on the skin, burning sensations, intense sensitivity, and chronic itching. Stretch marks are most frequently seen with *Bartonella* infections. Rashes resembling those found with broken blood vessels on the skin with dotted appearance happen more frequently with Babesiosis. There can also be flares of conditions that a patient had before contracting Lyme disease, such as seborrheic dermatitis and psoriasis. Typically, issues with skin, nails, and hair indicate issues with the hormone system. Almost every Lyme disease patient complains of problems in this area, with hair loss in women being the most frequent.

I have seen many symptoms involving hair, skin, and nails improve in patients when treated for Lyme disease using natural anti-inflammatories and addressing food sensitivities. Cycles of relapse and remission of tinea versicolor, a fungal infection of the skin that causes pigment loss, may also occur. For some, treatment of tick-borne disease results in a return of pigmentation to the skin. With patients who relapse, pigmentation diminishes again. This is another sign of the immune compromise that comes with a larger infection. Tinea versicolor is not contagious but will be more active during times of reduced internal vitality.

The three cardinal skin manifestations of Lyme disease are bull's-eye rash (erythema chronicum migrans), a painless bluish-red nodule or plaque (borrelial lymphocytoma), and red or bluish lesions progressing to atrophy of the skin, known as ACA (acrodermatitis chronica atrophicans).[25] Erythema migrans, the common bull's-eye rash, may appear days or weeks after tick attachment. It has become the key symptom used to determine if the bite was infectious, which can be misleading. Far too many people acquire Lyme disease without having developed a red ring at the site, so it should not be used as a confirmation. Borrelial lymphocytoma, which I have not seen in clinical practice, is one of the less common presentations. This symptom is more common with strains in Europe and looks like a red molelike swelling on the ear lobe or around the areola of the breast. With acrodermatitis chronica atrophicans, the skin can become thinner and darker in tone, with the skin looking aged beyond its years.

Lyme disease can trigger inflammatory responses in the body, altering the collagen matrix.[26] This creates weakness, with increased instability in tendons, ligaments, and skin. It alters the connective tissue within organ systems such as the heart and increases inflammation in the digestive tract, leading to inflammatory bowel disorders. Hyaluronic acid, a protein found in skin, joints, and ligaments, is impacted by the presence of spirochetes. This protein holds water in the tissues, allowing them to maintain lubrication and proper form. If the structure of these tissues is altered, they will dry out, leading to premature aging.

Calcifications and hypoxia (a deficiency in the amount of oxygen) also occur in joints and tendons, causing pain like that of carpal tunnel syndrome. Many patients present to the clinic with a history of surgery to correct carpal tunnel before they realized they may also have Lyme disease. They also experience more popping, cracking, and increased hypermobility of the joints. Hyaluronic acid can be supplemented by taking collagen type I/III and/or bone broth.

CARDIOVASCULAR AND RESPIRATORY SYSTEMS

Most patients in my office see a cardiologist before investigating Lyme disease. Typically, they are given a clean bill of health because the heart is normal according to all diagnostic testing, which includes electrocardiogram (EKG), echocardiogram, and stress tests. However, patients report heart palpitations, flutters, chest pain, rib pain, and low or high blood pressure. Shortness of breath can be a key symptom with *Babesia* infections, as are autonomic dysfunction and past history of asthma/allergies. Symptom flares in the cardiopulmonary system are the most common reason patients visit an emergency room—and for good reason, because heart attacks can be very subtle. It's always better to go to the emergency room than to stay home and risk an emergency. Typically, after being examined and tested at the emergency room, patients are discharged with antianxiety medications.

In more severe cases of Lyme disease, nerve conduction problems, called *bundle branch blocks*, can develop in the heart. This condition creates difficulty with proper heart rhythm and the contraction cycles responsible for adequately pumping blood through the heart. I have treated several patients over the years who have tick-borne disease with pericarditis, an infection and inflammation that develops in the fluid between the pericardium and the heart. This can constrict the heart because it reduces the space in which the heart can expand and contract with each beat. Fever may or may not accompany this infection, but pain is intense. Due to its critical nature, pericarditis requires medical management by a cardiovascular specialist who can monitor and medicate the condition as warranted. Patients who have issues with pericarditis also commonly have a confirmed diagnosis of Rocky Mountain spotted fever.

DIGESTIVE SYSTEM

Digestive issues are common patient complaints during their first office visit. These can include irritable bowel syndrome with alternating cycles of diarrhea and constipation, a recent onset of food allergy or intolerance, nausea, and/or changes in appetite leading to weight loss. Abdominal pain can vary from patient to patient, with some doubled over while others experience milder symptoms associated with gas and bloating. In children, abdominal pain is one of the primary symptoms of Lyme disease. Some patients have noted chronic burping as a symptom, but it's rare. Another interesting symptom mentioned over the years is the sensation of bugs crawling in the digestive tract.

Whatever the digestive complaint, the symptom requires support because the patient will need to tolerate oral medication. Whether natural or antibiotic, medications usually cause changes in digestive patterns. Patients with abdominal pain as part of a neurological component can be difficult to keep on medication because they may have what is known as a Herxheimer reaction (see chapter 6 for more on this response), which amplifies their pain and often leads them to discontinue the treatment.

Digestive distress related to Lyme disease is a combination of two issues: (1) increased inflammation in the gut, resulting in poor absorption and irritable bowel, and (2) increased sensitivity to foods.

Recently, I am often asked about tick-borne disease causing a red meat allergy. This is related to alpha-gal allergy, an anaphylactic reaction to a specific carbohydrate molecule found in the cells of animals that humans consume for food, such as cattle, pigs, and sheep. This allergic reaction can develop after the bite of a Lone Star tick, which, in the United States, most commonly carries ehrlichiosis or Rocky Mountain spotted fever. Other *Ixodes* species are implicated with the allergy in Australia and Europe. The alpha-gal allergic response usually involves itchy hives and gastrointestinal symptoms such as nausea two to six hours after ingesting red meat.

Gastroparesis is a neurological disorder that affects the rhythmic contractions of the intestinal tract. The digestive tract is often called the "second brain" because of the number of nerves centered there, required for gut motility, as well as the neurohormones that communicate with the brain. Lyme disease is known to cause inflammation in the nerve bundles that stimulate peristalsis. If the nerves in the gastrointestinal tract are affected by Lyme disease, gastric motility in the stomach can be altered. Though most people have milder forms of gastric distress such as constipation or nausea, severe gastroparesis can cause wasting due to the patient's inability to eat without severe abdominal pain.

One of the primary treatments for gastroparesis is intravenous Zithromax, a common intravenous medication used to treat tick-borne disease as well. While this medication treats the condition successfully, many in the medical community are reluctant to acknowledge that gastroparesis can have an infectious origin with Lyme disease. Patients with persistent digestive issues should also be worked up for food sensitivities, small intestinal bacterial overgrowth, parasite overgrowth, gastric emptying for delayed motility, and yeast overgrowth.

In Summary

The ability of the microbe to mobilize and migrate is the reason Lyme disease is so complicated. The most reliable attribute of Lyme disease is its lack of reliability in its presentation and response to treatment. Expect the unexpected. This infection can't be treated in a vacuum, managed by separate medical specialists each focusing on just one aspect of the body. This disease is multisystemic, requiring a holistic approach with a practitioner who understands its presentation in each organ system. Lyme disease is further complicated by the diversity of infections carried by the tick, each of which has its own unique set of symptoms.

In the next chapter, I'll give an overview of the coinfections commonly seen alongside Lyme disease. It's vital that coinfections be evaluated and treated to restore optimal health.

Fever

FEVERS ARE UNDERAPPRECIATED. It's a gift to be able to elevate our temperature to clear infections and toxins from our bodies. Yet our culture shuts fevers down with medication, either from fear of the possible deleterious effects of fever or because we allow ourselves little time to just recover. Deciding one's comfort level with allowing a fever to run its course is a personal choice, but fever will do more to clear an infection than any medication you could take. When we shut down a fever, we prolong the infection, not only for ourselves but for the larger population. Research has shown that people who use fever-reducing medications have a higher viral load and are more likely to spread the flu, even though their symptoms might be minimized to the point that they are functional enough to go to work. My personal process has been to let the fever go, as long as the patient can communicate clearly and drink water. Obviously, dehydration or a fever that goes beyond six or seven days would require more medical management.

Having been raised by a pharmacist, in a home where over-the-counter medication was always around for common ailments, I understand the cultural impulse to reduce the fever. But when I entered naturopathic medical school, I began to let go of the fear of fever. In fact, there were classes devoted to the practice of hydrotherapy, which includes a treatment called *hot fomentation*, in which body temperature is increased by using hot compresses and using wool blankets to wrap the patient like a burrito. This was helpful for those who hovered at a 99°F–100°F (37°C–38°C) fever without fully clearing the infection. The therapy could get the temperature high enough to provide momentum to resolve the infection.

Fever therapy is becoming better known, with a number of clinics in Europe offering it as a treatment. These clinics have been around for a long time, and their primary patient population is cancer patients. Recently, due to the increase in persistent chronic Lyme disease, the St. George Clinic in Germany has created protocols to medically induce fevers in a safe environment; vital signs, hydration status, and organ systems are monitored in a hospital setting while the body temperature is raised high enough for a proper duration to kill the pathogen. This treatment is currently not available in the United States due to FDA regulations.

CHAPTER 3

MORE THAN JUST LYME DISEASE: THE ROLE OF COINFECTIONS

A coinfection is the simultaneous infection of a host by more than one pathogen. It has become common to talk about the diverse population of microbes transmitted by a tick to a human as coinfections. A tick can carry several pathogens at one time as it collects them from mammals it feeds on. The next meal, a human, can be the recipient of not only the bacteria that carry Lyme disease but many other infections—and this can happen with just with one bite. Those who live in an area where ticks are endemic can have multiple tick bites over the course of years, increasing the body load of infections. Coinfections can be found at the time of a bite if the tick is sent out for testing. A tick may be carrying just one infection, such as anaplasmosis, which can cause rapid onset of headaches, neck pain, nausea, and fever. Because the environment in which ticks live has diverse flora and fauna, however, it's more realistic to expect more than one infection in the tick that bites you.

Be aware of the probability of coinfections so you can advocate for coinfection testing if Lyme disease is suspected. Comprehensive lab work to understand the infections present in your system is critical to finding the right treatment regimen (we will look at testing in chapter 4). Each infection has an affinity for certain tissue types, where disease will settle in; the infections can also cause overall immune deficiency. Many will lie dormant in lymphatic tissue, blood cells, nerves, and the walls of blood vessels. It's difficult for a body to fight Lyme disease if other bacterial, viral, or yeast infections or parasites are also depleting the body. We all carry infections we contracted in childhood or at other times of life, such as infections caused by the herpes family of viruses, and these add to the complexity of tick-borne illness.

Be aware of the probability of coinfections so you can advocate for coinfection testing if Lyme disease is suspected.

It's hard to say how many patients have coinfections because testing tends to be unreliable in capturing all of the infections, due to the variability of individual immune responses, strains for which testing may not be available, and the overlap of symptoms among the different infections. One of the most accurate ways to identify exposure to a coinfection is to test the tick, if it is found. TickReport (www.tickreport.com), a testing center affiliated with the University of Massachusetts, Amherst, publishes a Tick-borne Diseases Passive Surveillance list, which breaks down the rate of infection in the ticks tested. The database logs test results from tens of thousands of ticks collected since 2006 in the United States and Canada. The most prevalent positive infections found in the ticks collected, in order of highest to lowest rates, are *Borrelia burgdorferi*, anaplasmosis, and *Babesia* species.[1]

I find coinfection testing is frequently overlooked in the average primary care office. In my office, I request not only the Lyme disease Western blot, but also commercial lab testing for most of the common coinfection strains that can be idendified. If tests are positive, the infection is present; but if it's negative, it does not mean there is no infection—a confusing and frustrating concept. Most patients are diagnosed based on tick bite history, physical symptoms, and lab work. Sometimes the diagnosis is clear, and sometimes it is not. This is not always a comfortable place for patients or doctors to be.

An Act of Trust

Patients must take a leap of faith and trust a naturopathic doctor who diagnoses Lyme disease when the larger medical system does not seem to recognize the infection. If a patient is ill with all the signs of persistent infection, I'm doing my job as a doctor to treat that infection. I only do so if there is sufficient clinical evidence of infection, though; as I noted, negative lab results are not definitive. I must also rule out other conditions, such as autoimmune disease; however, these can be present simultaneously with tick-borne infections. Coinfections create a complex constellation of health issues for most patients. There is much debate about which infection is the primary one and which is the coinfection, and the way these infections manifest is highly individual. Tackling several infections can make the road to recovery very long, but healing is greatly improved when the patient stays open to the process and persists with treatment.

This overview breaks into categories—bacterial, viral, fungal, and parasitic—the infections commonly partnered with chronic Lyme disease. Information in this chapter is based on my clinical experience and research. The treatments discussed are merely options and are not limited to these examples. In most cases, both antibiotics and natural medications are required to recover fully from these infections. I list both forms because I use both in my practice.

Bacterial Coinfections

This section will guide you to a better understanding of the common bacterial coinfections seen in clinical practice. It's important to understand their chief indicators and typical symptoms in order to minimize fear: The most difficult aspect of tick-borne disease for patients is the fear associated with experiencing the unexplainable. These infections can have distinct presentations, almost like personality characteristics, which can be identified with specific symptoms; but patients are often told by doctors that what they are experiencing is not related to tick-borne infection. A better understanding of coinfections can help you identify your possible symptoms and know how to communicate your concerns to your providers.

BARTONELLOSIS

Of the more than twenty-six *Bartonella* species confirmed, the most infectious to humans are *B. henselae*, *B. quintana*, and *B. bacilliformis*. Bartonellosis is commonly associated with cat scratch fever. Often a localized skin infection that occurs after the bite or scratch from an infected cat, it can also become a systemic infection. This bacteria has been found in ticks in the United States, Europe, Asia, and the Middle East.[2] *B. quintana* primarily infects humans, whereas *B. henselae* is found in both humans and cats.[3] Cats acquire the disease from fleas and ticks.

Once the infection enters the human body, it infects red blood cells and the lining of vascular walls. The microbe itself has some ability to move through tissue, though not as efficiently as a spirochete. *Bartonella* produces an endotoxin while attaching to the interior of blood vessels with arm-like projections. Its presence stimulates inflammation in the body, which weakens vascular walls. The protein vascular endothelial growth factor (VEGF), a testable marker in the blood, is stimulated by *B. henslae*, increasing capillary growth in a condition called *angiogenesis*. This causes the growth of new vessels that are not necessary to the functioning of the body. Patients can rapidly develop capillaries under the skin, creating spider veins. Spider veins are not uncommon in those prone to them, but sudden onset is not common and should alert you to seek medical attention to address the cause. Part of the medical workup should be testing for *Bartonella* species.

The research on treatment for bartonellosis is all over the place, with some studies saying it's treatable and others claiming it is resistant to therapies. I have patients who improve with aggressive treatment, while other patients experience a prolonged and difficult recovery; but this is true of many infections. If not found early, *Bartonella* infections can require a lengthy recovery time, as is true of Lyme disease.

Symptoms: Among the most difficult symptoms of *Bartonella* are the mental and emotional changes; common behavioral changes include increased anger and obsessive-compulsive thinking. Patients may also tend toward addiction issues and violent thoughts. Mood-enhancing medications do not seem to work as well for those infected with *Bartonella*.[4] Patients often have a harder time reading and tracking information with their eyes and have many symptoms concerning visual acuity. They may be more sensitive to light, see flashes of light in their field of vision, and have eye pain and/or blurred vision.

For school-age patients, grades will suffer and they may experience a loss of confidence. Those who have bartonellosis may also be diagnosed with attention deficit, show autism spectrum–like behaviors where there were none before, or demonstrate hyperactivity or antisocial behaviors. Other common complaints are numbness and tingling, shooting pains, electrical shock sensations, vibrations down the extremities, enlarged lymph nodes, lumps forming under the skin, walking abnormalities, inflammation in the heart muscle, intense pain, weakness in the lower limbs, loss of muscle tone, hypermobility mimicking Ehlers-Danlos syndrome type II, rashes, and behavioral changes.[5]

All sort of rashes may appear with bartonellosis. Random lines may show up in areas where no skin contact created them. Or the rash can look like stretch marks, with gender-specific patterning: males have lines across the back in a horizontal pattern, while females typically have them around the armpits, hips, and down the thighs. These are present in cases where there is no associated weight gain that would cause the marks. A chicken wire pattern on the skin or dramatic changes in skin color with intense red and purples may occur, with the skin then returning to normal. Other symptoms include clusters of capillaries that appear randomly, sprouting up overnight; poorer circulation and a condition called *Raynaud's syndrome*; low-grade fevers that come and go throughout the day; enlarged lymph nodes throughout the body that enlarge and shrink in a chronic cycle; and burning sensations in the limbs and mouth.

Blood tends to be thicker in those with bartonellosis, and the vascular system is affected due to an immune response that causes excess proteins to be created. Blood can appear like syrup, witnessed when taking a blood draw—this is obvious, as it takes longer for the tubes to fill. Patients have increased pain due to the poor circulation caused by the blood vessel injuries and thicker blood. Natural or pharmaceutical blood thinner can be of assistance here, with proper medical management.

Treatment options: *Pharmaceutical medications*—sulfamethoxazole-trimethoprim (Bactrim), rifampin, doxycycline/minocycline

Natural treatments—Houttuynia, gou teng (*Unicaria rhyncophylla*), L-arginine, garlic, pokeroot, sarsaparilla, *Angelica sinensis*, skullcap, cordyceps, glucosamine, white peony root, kudzu. For blood thinning and endothelial repair: nattokinase, fish oil, lumbrokinase, serrapeptase, bromelain, quercetin, resveratrol

EHRLICHIOSIS/ANAPLASMOSIS

Human monocytic ehrlichiosis and human granulocytic anaplasmosis are very similar in their presentation. Their primary cellular targets are monocytes, macrophages, and leukocytes, which are all part of the family of white blood cells. These bacteria enter the white blood cell and reprogram it to serve the bacteria's purpose of survival.[6] Our immune system has a difficult time with this change, which allows other fungal, parasitic, viral, or additional bacterial infections to become more problematic.

The good news is that these infections are highly treatable. Ehrlichiosis is noted to be transmitted by the Lone Star tick, and anaplasmosis by the deer tick, *Ixodes scapularis*. Ehrlichiosis is most commonly found in Mississippi, Oklahoma, Tennessee, Arkansas, and Maryland. I have seen many patients with positive ticks in New Hampshire and Massachusetts as well. Anaplasmosis is primarily found in New England and the north central United States.

Symptoms: Ehrlichiosis and anaplasmosis are infections with a rapid onset, causing people to seek medical care immediately. Typically, within a day or two of the bite, patients run a high fever (103°F–105°F [39°C–41°C]). Then neck pain, respiratory issues, elevated liver enzymes, headaches, muscle pain, joint pain, rashes (specifically with ehrlichiosis), abdominal pain, nausea, and vomiting follow. Meningitis and encephalitis are also common and require in-hospital medical care. Nerve involvement may also occur, with facial palsy and loss of sensation in different parts of the body. There can be inflammation within organ tissues, including in the spleen, kidneys, and heart.

Many patients are diagnosed with viral meningitis, as the presentation of fever, intense neck pain, nausea, and headache is similar. Ehrlichiosis and anaplasmosis may not be tested if a viral cause is assumed. The patient is usually cared for in a hospital setting, given fluids and medical support until the symptoms improve enough for the patient to be released. However, as time goes by, the patient reports relapses, with continued body pain, headaches, and cognition and neurological issues because they are actually suffering from a bacterial infection that requires treatment with antibiotics.

Treatment options: *Pharmaceutical medications*—doxycycline/minocycline, rifampin

Natural treatments—Sho-saiko-to, reishi, Maitake Gold Fraction, green tea extract, arabinogalactan, elderberry, olive leaf extract, liposomal glutathione, artichoke, milk thistle

ROCKY MOUNTAIN SPOTTED FEVER

Telling a patient he is positive for Rocky Mountain spotted fever (RMSF) is very difficult because the first thing you see when you jump online to research this disease is "death." I do not wish to downplay the severity of the RMSF, but I see patients test for this disease, caused by the bacterium *Rickettsia rickettsii*, at least two or three times a week. Most patients will be Lyme disease positive as well. I treat patients aggressively and see titers decrease within two to three months' time.

RMSF is considered one of the most commonly acquired and lethal *Rickettsia* infections in the United States. It's transmitted by a variety of tick vectors in the United States, including the American dog tick (*Dermacentor variabilis*), the American wood tick (*Dermacentor andersoni*), and the brown dog tick (*Rhipicephalus sanguineus*). Other *Rickettsia* infections are *R. parkeri*, *R. phillipi*, *R. massiliae*, and possibly *R. montanensis* and *R. amblyommii*.[7] While RMSF is regarded as more prevalent in southern U.S. states, most of my patients who are positive have never visited the South. A lot of current research is focused on RMSF in Mexico.

In the body, RMSF is an intracellular bacterial infection that invades blood vessels of medium size.[8] Patients typically experience symptoms four to ten days after a tick bite; tick attachment time is four to ten hours to transmit disease. As with Lyme disease, proteins within tick saliva can boost transmission of the infection.[9]

Symptoms: New infections commonly present with headaches, fevers, chills, nausea, and abdominal pain. If the disease becomes chronic, mental confusion, hepatitis, cardiovascular inflammation, and rashes on the arms/legs can also occur. Neurological manifestations include altered gait, short-term memory loss, stuttering, sensitivity to light, and emotional instability.

Treatment options: *Pharmaceutical medications*—doxycycline/minocycline and rifampin. Tetracycline medications are not indicated typically until after the age of eight to ten years. The use of medications in the tetracycline family can cause softening of the teeth, which alters adult dentition. I have seen improvement with the use of sulfa medications in young children, even though the literature does not support this at this time. The recommended treatment time in the literature is seven to ten days; however, I usually treat longer, until symptoms are resolved. Because of the severity of the antibiotic medication, I strongly recommend that natural medication support be implemented as well.

Natural treatments—resveratrol, olive leaf extract, quercetin, horse chestnut, hesperidin, rutin, lomatium, cryptolepis, and gou teng (*Unicaria rhyncophylla*). My recommendation is to use natural medicine in conjunction with prescription medications rather than alone, due to the risk of complications. The goal is to treat the vascular system and the immune system.

Q FEVER

Discovered in Australia in 1937, Q fever is also known as *Coxiella burnetii,* or query fever. It's prominent in the United States, the tropics, the Netherlands, and the Middle East. A small intracellular bacterium shaped like a ball, *Coxiella burnetii* is highly adaptable to stressful situations in the body. It has a dense, interwoven structure, which helps it maintain stability. These bacteria can survive for seven to ten months in wool garments at ambient temperature, for more than one month on fresh meat, and for more than forty months in milk.[10] They have also been known to survive in low concentrations of formaldehyde solution, a common preservative for tissue samples. The take-home is that it's a survivor. The good news is that it does seem to be susceptible to antibiotics.

The most common modes of transmission are from inhalation of particles of amniotic fluid after birth of new livestock, tick bites, and ingesting food that harbors the bacteria. The main reservoirs are cattle, sheep, and goats.

Ticks were first recognized as a reservoir in Montana in the hard-bodied tick species *D. andersoni. C. burnetii* has since been found in forty different hard-bodied tick species, several soft-bodied tick species, flies, mites, and bed bugs.[11] The microbe lives in the gut, salivary glands, and ovaries of the tick species for long periods of time. The stress on the tick—dehydration and minimal feeding—does not seem to affect the presence of infection. Q fever can be found in tick feces as well. Ticks collected in an urban park in Italy were found to have a triple coinfection of *Rickettsia* species, *B. burgdorferi* species, and *C. burnetii*.[12] This result underscores my earlier note that the most effective way to determine infectivity is by testing the ticks.

Symptoms: Q fever can last up to fourteen days in acute form and may also persist as a long-term chronic infection. Its initial symptoms are fevers, headaches, fatigue, and muscle pain, with more severe symptoms including endocarditis, hepatitis, meningitis, pneumonia, and chronic fatigue. Older men tend to be more symptomatic than women. Severe complications in pregnancy and childbirth can occur, with the infection able to replicate in the placenta. This can cause many birth complications and abnormal development of the fetus. Even after the baby is born, the infection can stay in the mother's body and infect the next pregnancy if she is not treated.[13]

When contracted in childhood, the disease is less symptomatic than it is in adults. It can look like a common cold. High fevers can last more than fifteen days; other symptoms include cough, joint pain, muscle pain, abdominal pain, nausea, severe headaches, elevated liver enzymes, Guillain-Barré syndrome, peripheral neuropathy, rashes, enlarged lymph nodes, elevated autoimmune markers in blood, and chest pain with breathing.

Treatment options: *Pharmaceutical medications*—doxycycline/minocycline plus hydroxychloroquine, sulfamethoxazole-trimethoprim

Natural treatments—olive leaf extract, garlic, lomatium, *Sida acuta*, goldenseal, Oregon grape root, Hoxsey-like formula, homeopathic nosode of Q fever

FRANCISELLA TULAREMIA

Infection with *Francisella tularensis* is commonly known as *rabbit fever*, with the primary vector being cottontail rabbits and hares. This disease saw a peak of infectivity in the early 1900s, with some outbreaks in North America in the 1980s and early 2000s. The bacteria are transmitted via ticks and biting flies, but can also be contracted if a person consumes infected food or water or inhales particles in the air. The infection typically has a quick onset of two to six days but can take up to twenty-one days to manifest.

Symptoms: New infection presents with fever, rashes, nausea, muscle pain, cough, vomiting, sore throat, enlarged lymph nodes in the neck, abdominal pain, and pneumonia-like symptoms. There can be an ulcerative lesion at the site of the bite, with lymph node involvement.

Treatment options: *Pharmaceutical medications*—intravenous gentamicin, intramuscular streptomycin, and oral doxycycline

Natural treatments—olive leaf extract, garlic, lomatium, *Sida acuta*, goldenseal, Oregon grape root, Hoxsey-like formula, Maitake Gold Fraction, green tea extract

Other Bacterial Infections

While *Mycoplasma* pneumonia and *Chlamydia* pneumonia are commonly passed around within the human and animal population, peer-reviewed studies have shown the prevalence of both infections within ticks of the *Ixodes* species. A study published in *Applied Environmental Microbiology* in 2015 used DNA sequencing to find proof of *Chlamydia* species with ticks.[14] *Mycobacterium* species were determined to be the cause of body pain, fatigue, and cognitive issues without any other sign of Lyme disease soon after a tick bite. After treatment for *Mycoplasma*, symptoms abated.[15] There is so much we do not know about what ticks carry and transmit. Investigating the presence of these two infections is important in symptom management and recovery.

MYCOPLASMA PNEUMONIA

Mycoplasma pneumonia, sometimes called *walking pneumonia*, is a common finding on patients' lab results, showing that a majority of my patients have been exposed at some point in their lives. Most of the time, *Mycoplasma* pneumonia presents with antibodies signaling past infection rather than as a current acute disease. Common in the human population, this infection is typically transmitted from human to human through contact with respiratory fluids. It tends to cycle through the population every five to seven years but can have a decades-long incubation period before it reemerges. It's a very small bacterium that adheres to respiratory tissue and requires our cholesterol for survival, and its cell structure can make certain antibiotics less effective. This type of pneumonia can be severe enough to cause hospitalization or so mild that its main symptom is a persistent cough.

Mycoplasma pneumoniae is important to consider in conjunction with chronic Lyme disease because infection with this bacterium creates a more difficult recovery for someone with Lyme, as the coinfection can cause breathing difficulty, fatigue, muscle pain, and, for some reason, a high propensity for hair loss in women.

Symptoms: *Mycoplasma* pneumonia can cause chronic arthritic and neurological symptoms, and is a cofactor in developing rheumatoid arthritis[16] as well. Joints affected are knees, shoulders, elbows, and wrists, which will be swollen and warm to touch. This is thought to be due to direct exposure to the microbial toxins, which cause an immune reaction in the host and lead to tissue damage. Nervous system involvement usually starts with respiratory infection, with the most common manifestation being inflammation around the brain and the nerves throughout the body. The eyes are also affected, with increased risk of optic neuritis or double vision.[17] It is important to check the active status of this infection in those who may have tick-borne disease, especially if the person is short of breath or has a persistent cough.

Mycoplasma pneumonia can lead to a chronic cough that lasts months or years as well as an increased risk of developing asthma. It also comes with increased risk of severe skin reactions, hemolytic anemia, or severely low platelets. This infection has also been associated with inflammatory bowel disease[18] and Crohn's disease.[19]

Treatment options: *Pharmaceutical medications*—tetracycline and macrolides. Does not respond to rifampin, penicillins, cephalosporins, or sulfonamides.

Natural treatments—olive leaf, lomatium, garlic, elderberry, bromelain. Natural expectorants are *N*-acetyl-cysteine (NAC), bromelain, and guaifenesin. For persistent cough, use Old English Ivy tincture or thyme tea. Herbals that support neurological tissue such as bacopa, phosphatidylcholine, turmeric, tianma (*Gastrodia elata Blume*), gou teng (*Unicaria rhynocophylla*), yarrow, *Rhodiola rosea*.

CHLAMYDIA PNEUMONIA

Commonly acquired in childhood, *Chlamydia* pneumonia can persist into adulthood when the person's immune system is compromised. This is a common infection to test when Lyme disease is present, to get an understanding of bacterial load that might make recovery more complicated. These bacteria behave in the body like parasites; they are taken into a host's immune cells and use the host cell energy to survive. Most bacteria require amino acids to survive, and *Chlamydia pneumoniae* is no different. The infection does best when the amino acids we rely on for maintaining proper health, such as methionine or lysine, are low.[20]

Chlamydia pneumonia is a very common infection, affecting 50 percent of the population, with acute infection affecting mostly young people. Men seem to be affected more than women. Humans are the primary reservoir, passing the infection through mucous droplets released in the air. This is a concomitant infection, meaning that it occurs or exists at the same time as another infection, and it is enhanced by other systemic infections such as Lyme disease. A patient can carry the disease and be asymptomatic, but it will resurface if person's immunity is reduced.

Symptoms: pharyngitis, sinusitis, cough, fever, hoarse voice; associated with increased risk of coronary artery disease, sarcoidosis, asthma, and reactive arthritis

Treatment options: *Pharmaceutical medications*—macrolides and doxycyline/minocycline

Natural treatments—lysine and methionine, elderberry, cordyceps, Maitake Gold D-fraction, astragalus, bromelain, reishi, *N*-acetyl-cysteine (NAC)

Microbial Diversity in Ticks

THERE ARE MORE UNKNOWNS THAN KNOWNS when it comes to tick bites. I always warn patients not to get too fixated on Lyme disease—unfortunately, *Borrelia* species are far from the only pathogens ticks carry. Tick microbiomes, like those of humans, are incredibly biodiverse; and we are just beginning to understand how varied a tick is as we sequence its genome. If a tick is carrying multiple microbes, it is nearly impossible for Lyme spirochetes to be the only microbe transmitted. In fact, when larval ticks fed from mice treated with gentamicin (an antibiotic), they went through *dysbiosis*, which slowed their interest in feeding quite dramatically.[21] This is similar to the cravings or changes in appetite we humans face when our microbes are altered.

By understanding the pathogens in the ticks found in a given area, we can attempt to stay on top of diseases that could eventually make their way into the human population instead of chasing infections after the fact. As the climate continues to change, leading to longer spring/autumn seasons, and the environment is less agricultural and more urbanized, ticks will migrate farther north and have longer periods of high activity. Because the tick microbiome is dependent on geographical location, the tick will be introduced to new infections.

Other factors also affect the tick microbiome, including gender—male ticks have more genetic variation in their microbiomes than female ticks. Thankfully, a majority of the microbes in the tick midgut are nonpathogenic, just as in the human microbiome.

Ongoing research is looking at the tick immune system and its microbiome in relation to the microbes being transmitted and how coinfections emerging in endemic areas behave within the tick.

Viral Coinfections

There are more viral proteins on the planet than any other microbe. It's important to investigate these infections with testing because their opportunistic nature and ability to increase inflammation markers in the body make it difficult for a person with both a viral infection and Lyme disease to regain health. Following is an overview of the most common viral infections tested for and commonly treated in my clinic. When I say treated, I mean that we offer medications to slow replication of the virus, not that we cure it. Viruses are with us for life.

Viruses persist by replicating virions, which infect cells. Virions are programmed proteins floating freely in the environment, like multitudes of USB drives floating in space. They then plug themselves into the cellular membrane of a compatible cell, and the data are uploaded into the RNA/DNA of the cell. This new information causes our DNA, the program model for our cells, to change cell structure and behavior. These changes can create discomfort in the body in the form of illness, but in many cases these data support life on the planet through the sharing of information. For example, a virus is responsible for the expression of the protein syncytin, which helps in creating a healthy placenta for the growth and development of fetuses in mammals, humans included.[22] When we hear the word *virus*, we think of illness and suffering, but viruses have been here since the beginning of life on the planet. The data they carry are far vaster than we can imagine and benefit our survival by educating our bodies to adapt to the ever-changing environment.

As part of an initial assessment of a patient, I check titers for the common viral infections herpes simplex virus I/II, Epstein-Barr, cytomegalovirus, parvovirus, and human herpesvirus 6. Viral replication can increase when the body is run-down with other infections. Recovery from Lyme disease will be more difficult if these viruses are not addressed.

Because the treatment for viruses is the same in each case, I am including the options here rather than for each virus separately.

Treatment options: *Pharmaceutical medications*—valacyclovir and acyclovir

Natural treatments—Lemon balm, L-lysine, propolis, *Andrographis paniculata*, *Astragalus membranaceus*, *Houttuynia cordata*, olive leaf extract, vitamin A, lomatium, cryptolepis, garlic, Maitake Gold Fraction, goldenseal, oregano oil, neem, vitamin C, *Polygonum cuspidatum*, *Scutterlaria*, phosphatidylcholine, medium-chain triglycerides

POWASSAN VIRUS (TICK-BORNE ENCEPHALITIS)

Powassan virus was first found in a young boy in Powassan, Ontario, in 1958 and is the only tick-borne encephalitis in the United States. It's transmitted by *Ixodes scapularis* in the northeastern United States and *Ixodes cookei* in the Midwest and Canada. Transmission can occur within three hours of a person receiving a tick bite. Tick saliva enhances the transmission of the viral infection, which shows an affinity for the brain tissues and causes inflammation in the brain, leading to meningoencephalitis, encephalitis, and aseptic meningitis.[23] This virus has been found in Europe and Canada and has been confirmed in New York and Pennsylvania; there has been a 671 percent rise in this infection over the past eighteen years.[24]

Tick-borne encephalitis is more prevalent in Russia and Europe, with 10,000 to 13,000 cases confirmed in those regions annually,[25] with 90 percent

Herpesviruses are opportunistic infections that replicate more aggressively when the body's vitality is weakened ...

developing flulike symptoms and the other 10 percent developing more severe neurological manifestations.[26] A vaccination is available for forms of tick-borne encephalitis found in Eastern Europe and Russia, but there is no formal treatment for Powassan/tick-borne encephalitis. The primary focus is symptoms management at the time of acute onset, with hydration, pain management, anti-inflammatories, antivirals, and steroids. Ongoing neurological deficits can occur and can ideally be managed by natural medications to enhance immunity and reduce neuroinflammation.

Symptoms: Infection of the brain and meningitis. Usually, intense headaches, high fevers around 105°F–106°F (41°C), nausea, intense neck pain, altered speech, loss of limb function, memory loss, and seizures are among the symptoms of Powassan virus and tick-borne encephalitis.

HERPESVIRUSES

There are eight herpesviruses infectious to humans. These are classified into three categories: alpha-herpesviruses, beta-herpesviruses, and gamma-herpesviruses. Alpha-herpesviruses are quick replicators and include oral herpes (herpes simplex virus I), genital herpes (herpes simplex virus II), and chicken pox (varicella zoster). Beta-herpesviruses include cytomegaloviruses and human herpesvirus 6, which are slower to replicate. The gamma-herpesvirus that most concerns Lyme disease patients is Epstein-Barr virus, which acts almost like a parasite, infecting 6.5 billion people around the world. Herpesviruses have been traced back over two hundred million years.[27]

Herpesviruses seem to have an affinity for nerve tissue and specific cells of the immune system. When borne by ticks, each of these infections has similarities of presentation, including fatigue, nerve pain, rashes, sweats, muscle pain, and fevers. Herpesviruses are opportunistic infections that replicate more aggressively when the body's vitality is weakened, and viral replication becomes more active in someone who is experiencing chronic Lyme disease, making recovery more difficult. It's important to test for these infections and treat them at the same time other tick-borne infections are addressed with natural antiviral medication and, if necessary, prescription antivirals. In clinical settings, doctors are more likely to test for Epstein-Barr or other herpes viral infections, assuming the patient only has a virus when he actually has Lyme disease. In most cases, both are present.

Cytomegalovirus (CMV)

Cytomegalovirus (CMV), or human herpesvirus 5, poses the greatest difficulty for newborns and those who are immunocompromised. Symptoms in this population can include liver and spleen involvement, rashes, and inflammation of the retina, blood vessel walls, and the smooth muscle of the kidneys. These symptoms especially affect those with lower levels of an important immune cell type called *natural killer cells*, which are cells that attack a foreign invader immediately after it enters the body. They are our first line of defense.

CMV can go into long periods of inactivity, reemerging when it senses the body is in a state of compromise and stress. It also has the ability to reprogram lymphocytes—a type of white blood cell that is part of the immune system— to dissuade them from attacking.[28] As cells are invaded by the virus, they can appear larger, hence the name *cytomegalovirus*. It's also associated with Guillain-Barré symptoms and peripheral neuropathic pain.

There is an interesting dynamic in the relationship between cytomegalovirus and multiple sclerosis (MS). We typically believe that viruses are harmful to our health; however, researchers have hypothesized that CMV is immune-protective with regard to MS. Reduced MS symptoms and the presence of CMV are strongly correlated in MS patients.[29] This could represent a breakthrough, leading to more research on the benefits some viruses may yield.

Symptoms: Symptoms can be barely perceivable when the disease is acquired, with slight lymph node enlargement, low fever, and fatigue. A hallmark of the disease is relapse and remission cycles, in which the disease is shed in tears, sweat, blood, urine, semen, and breast milk. The disease is transmitted when body fluids of an infected person come in contact with the mucous membranes of another. Congenital transmission can cause hearing loss, visual impairments, seizures, and mental/physical disabilities in immunocompromised infants. Risk factors in adults with CMV and other diseases that compromise the immune system, such as Lyme disease, can be hepatitis, enlarged spleen, pneumonia, and encephalitis.

Herpes Simplex Virus I and II

With herpes simplex virus I and II, lesions are typically found on the surface of the skin around the mouth and genitals. Initially, an acute crop of lesions appears together with nerve pain. This is when it is most contagious, spread from person to person with direct skin contact. Blood work and swabs from new lesions can confirm the strain of infection. Although it's commonly assumed that herpes type I only creates lesions on the mouth, it can cause genital herpes as well. Herpes I and II have an affinity for sensory nerves, where they can go dormant, reemerging during times of stress.

Herpes simplex has been associated with encephalitis and inflammation in the temporal lobes of the brain. It can also cause headaches, fevers, and changes in speech and behavior.[30] The skin lesions can continue to flare, brought on by stress and/or dietary triggers such as foods high in L-arginine (including coffee, cheese, and red wine). Herpes simplex is transmitted with skin-to-skin contact when an infected person has an active lesion. Individuals with herpes type I/II will have more superficial outbreaks after acquiring Lyme disease, though they might have gone years without having an active infection. Again, this is due to compromise of the immune system.

Symptoms: Nerve pain, headaches, fevers, lesions that can be oral as well as genital, with initial tingling or burning at the site before the lesions fully manifest. There can also be intense pain at the site of the lesions, ear pain, and facial palsy. The reactivation of herpes simplex virus can complicate the picture for Lyme disease with nerve pain and lymph node involvement. Herpes simplex virus also can cause vagus nerve palsies or temporary paralysis, leading to difficulty swallowing and speaking clearly.

Human Herpes Virus 6 (HHV-6)

Human herpesvirus 6 (HHV-6) infection, commonly referred to as *roseola*, is contracted early in childhood, between the ages of six months and twenty-four months. It's characterized by a "slapped cheek" appearance, with a red, raised rash that appears after a high fever; irritability; and ear pain. It can also cause febrile seizures, which can happen when fevers are too high, but seizures have not been found to be linked to the development of more severe forms of epilepsy. A reactivation of HHV-6 in an adult can be linked to encephalitis or meningitis.[31] HHV-6 has also been found postmortem in the brain tissue of individuals with MS and is theorized as a contributor in the progression of the disease. HHV-6 is diagnosed after the virus is identified in cerebrospinal fluid. This test is most commonly run in patients suffering from symptoms of encephalitis. It will also attack specific cells of the immune system, including microglial cells of the brain, lymphocytes, and natural killer cells.

Symptoms: Chronic fatigue syndrome or mononucleosis-like symptoms, abdominal discomfort, upper respiratory infection, chronic enlarged lymph nodes, anemia, arthritis, rashes, irritability, thyroid dysfunction, and peripheral neuropathies. The majority of people who carry this virus present with no symptoms at all.

Epstein-Barr Virus

Just about every patient, regardless of whether he has Lyme disease, has been exposed to Epstein-Barr virus, with more than six billion infected people on the planet. A majority of my patients have positive titers for Epstein-Barr, with a majority experiencing chronic active Epstein-Barr syndrome. I test all patients, not to evaluate whether they have the virus but to get a baseline of their titers. It's weird if someone is negative, and it leaves me wondering how they escaped such a common viral infection.

Epstein-Barr virus will reactivate when the body is under stress from other diseases or life situations. Known as *mononucleosis*, the more pronounced form of Epstein-Barr is also referred to as the "kissing disease" because of its affinity for the tonsils, which allow it to be transmitted in saliva. It likes to make its home in the lymphocytes (white blood cells) and lymphatic tissue (tonsils) and has been linked to an increased risk of developing certain forms of cancers, or lymphomas.

Just about every patient, regardless of whether he has Lyme disease, has been exposed to Epstein-Barr virus, with more than six billion infected people on the planet.

Research published in *Nature Genetics* in 2018 found that Epstein-Barr virus increased a person's risk of developing lupus, rheumatoid arthritis, inflammatory bowel disease, type 1 diabetes, and celiac disease.[32] The interaction of Epstein-Barr with the human immune system alters gene expression, increasing the likelihood that an individual will develop one or more of the conditions. It can also cause the myelin around nerves to degrade, creating numbness and tingling throughout the body due to chronic inflammation.[33]

Frequently, patients have both mononucleosis and a positive Western blot for Lyme disease. This can be confusing because mononucleosis can cause swollen glands, fevers, muscle pain, debilitating fatigue, and sweats—but so can Lyme disease. Mononucleosis is diagnosed more often because it's more readily tested in conventional clinical settings. If the confirmatory test for mononucleosis is negative, the diagnosis is often subclinical mono, and the patient is sent home to rest and recuperate with no further testing. Many patients are treated with immunosuppressant steroids, which, in my opinion, is the worst medication to give at a time the immune system is trying to fight an infection. The bottom line is that everyone should be tested for Epstein-Barr and levels of antibodies tracked on labs to check how much the virus is contributing to the patient's ill health.

Symptoms: Fatigue, fever, loss of appetite, rashes, sore throat, enlarged lymph nodes, enlarged spleen, increased inflammation markers referred to as *unbalanced cytokine response*,[34] night sweats, and low natural killer cell counts.

Varicella Zoster

Varicella zoster, or chicken pox, is a virus transmitted by direct contact or by droplets of mucus breathed into the air by an infected person. Later in life, this virus can resurface as shingles, or herpes zoster. Before the vaccine was available, nearly everyone got chicken pox, and parents went out of their way to have their children infected just to get it over with. When children are infected, they typically recover within a couple of weeks, whereas those who are first infected in adulthood can become more severely ill. I do not often see shingles in my office, yet patients do report a history of having had it in the past.

Symptoms: Headaches, fever, malaise, and rash over the entire body lasting two to three weeks, usually in childhood. Later in adulthood, patients can develop multiple vesicles with blisterlike presentation along a sensory nerve root or a dermatome. These can be weeping and then crust over to heal within one to two weeks' time. This usually follows a stressful event or another illness that causes immune compromise. These can form anywhere on the body but are most common along the waistline or on the trunk of the body on one side. Outbreaks can also occur on the hands, with pain and vesicles called *herpetic whitlow*. This virus, over time, can lead to immune compromise.

HUMAN PARVOVIRUS B19

Human parvovirus B19 was discovered in 1974. It's the only infection in the parvovirus family that is pathogenic to humans; another type of parvovirus is well known as a canine infection. Parvovirus B19, also known as *fifth disease*, is transmitted by droplets in the air, via blood, or from mother to baby. In children ages one to five, the virus begins with a fever and ends with a rash. This virus becomes more problematic if it's transmitted in utero, as it has the potential to cause miscarriage due to infection of the placenta.

In chronic persisting infections, there can be symmetrical swelling of joints, which is typically seen in rheumatoid arthritis. It can also cause aplastic anemia, a condition in which the body temporarily stops making red blood cells. Parvovirus B19 should be considered as a potential additional cause when joint swelling with symmetrical appearance occurs in those with Lyme disease; often, this is mistakenly diagnosed as rheumatoid arthritis.

Symptoms: In early childhood, parvovirus B19 is referred to as "slapped cheek" disease due to the facial rash. Common symptoms in youth are fever, upset stomach, headache, and runny nose. Blood work shows anemia. The virus can also cause arthritis and can look a lot like Lyme disease arthritis. The viral timing is spring and winter, with joint manifestation happening a few weeks after infection, coinciding with ticks' more active periods in endemic areas. There can be increased swelling in the joint as well as morning stiffness similar to osteoarthritis.

Fungal Coinfections

Commonly seen as unappealing, funguses are often associated with disease. However, some funguses are becoming more widely admired for their complex communication networks and other qualities—such as the ability to eat plastics—that could be helpful on a global scale. This section, however, focuses on the pathogenic *Candida* (yeast) species that colonize the skin and mucosal surfaces in cases of immune compromise.

Mucosal surfaces are those that are more pink, sensitive, and lubricated, such as the oral cavity, sinus cavity, vaginal canal, and digestive tract. This differs from outer skin surfaces and nails, which have a protein called *keratin* that creates a strong barrier on the outside. This barrier can withstand friction and temperature changes, and is waterproof. *Candida* can colonize internally or externally, but other skin fungal infections—including those caused by dermatophytes or *Tinea* species—colonize the keratinized tissues. These infections include ringworm and nail fungus.

Funguses such as *Candida albicans* are present within the healthy human flora and can be introduced into the body when a person eats contaminated food. Funguses such as *Aspergillus* species can be inhaled through spores in the air in certain areas of the country. Dermatophytes are acquired externally by physical contact with the skin of the foot, such as when a person walks on the floor of a shared gym shower.

Opportunistic yeast species pathogenic to humans include *C. albicans* and *C. glabrata*, but there are more than two hundred species of yeast.[35] Only certain strains can exist in the gut, which has low oxygen and a temperature too high for most strains. Part of the normal gut flora, yeast can get out of balance when a person's immune system is compromised due to infection, toxic overload, or improper diet. The *Candida* cell looks like an oval, and when it reproduces (asexually), a bud extends off its body and is eventually released as a new yeast cell. Yeast loves sugar and thrives in areas where the pH does not support healthy growth of *Lactobacillus* and *Bifidobacterium* species, two of the most prolific beneficial bacterial strains in the body that help maintain healthy yeast population numbers. Yeast can also create biofilm slime, which I talked about in chapter 2.

Symptoms: Clinical presentations depend on the area affected. Many patients have a history of repeated vaginal yeast infections or athlete's foot.

Outer skin manifestations of yeast imbalance can be redness, often called a "red, beefy rash," cracked skin, peeling, itching, and darker skin patches that look like dry circles with a tan appearance. Some dermatophytes of the skin are slow growing and are difficult to treat, especially nail fungus. Areas commonly affected are skin folds, such as those in the groin, armpits, under breasts, and in the abdomens of those with more abdominal fat stores. This is because skin folds tend to have the higher moisture content yeast like. Feet are also common sites of fungal infections because they are in shoes throughout the day. Symptoms of vaginal yeast infections are itching, redness, and discharge. Sinus infections caused by yeast tend to be more persistent because it is not common to swab the nasal cavity to check for yeast; it is assumed the infection is bacterial, viral, or allergen driven.

Treatment options: *Pharmaceutical medications*—topical creams such as clotrimazole, fluconazole, and miconazole available over the counter; oral treatment of nystatin and fluconazole; intravenous amphotericin B

Natural treatments—monolaurin, neem, *Saccharomyces boulardii*, gentian violet, pau d'arco, caprylic acid, oregano oil, berberine-containing herbs, probiotics, allicin (garlic), and *Pseudowintera colorata* (topical Kolorex?)

Parasitic Coinfections

A parasite is an entity dependent on another being that does not provide a benefit to the host. Almost everyone has a gastrointestinal parasite, which is not a problem unless it creates digestive distress such as diarrhea, bloating, weight loss, or malabsorption of nutrients (which means malabsorption of medications as well). Parasites infectious to humans fall into two categories: protozoa and helminths. I'll talk about protozoa first, then tackle helminths a bit later.

Protozoa are single-cell organisms that move from host to host through an oral–fecal route, usually through contaminated food, tainted water, or intimate human contact. They can also be spread by blood-sucking insects, as with the infection babesiosis. The infections most commonly seen in humans are giardiasis, cryptosporidiosis, amebiasis (from *Entamoeba histolytica*), and malaria (from *Plasmodium* species). Protozoa have erratic growth cycles, making them difficult to catch in stool analysis. Depending on the species, they can produce many offspring. Usually, two or three random samples of stool are required to increase likelihood of identifying them.

BABESIOSIS

Babesia species are protozoal single-cell parasites transmitted by ticks. Babesiosis is related to malaria, which is carried by mosquitos. *Babesia* have an affinity for red blood cells and are referred to as piroplasms because of their pear shape within the red blood cell, visible with blood smear tests.

They are one of the most prevalent blood parasites in the world, initially identified by Romanian scientist Victor Babes in 1888, when several cattle were infected.

Ixodes ticks are the only ones known to carry babesiosis. There have been more than one hundred *Babesia* species identified, with only a small percentage of those causing illness in humans. Studies have shown that 40–60 percent of white-footed mice are infected with *B. microti*, which infects ticks in the nymph stage.[36] However, birds and rodents alike can be reservoirs for the infection. *B. duncani* WA-1 was first identified in patients in Washington State, so many practitioners feel that it is a West Coast disease; but I see a large number of positive tests in New England in patients who have never been out West.[37]

Because of *Babesia*'s parasitic relationship with red blood cells, the cells' ability to carry oxygen and retrieve cellular wastes is negatively affected. Red blood cells are often discarded by the body and sent to the spleen, which leads to swelling and pain in this organ, along the lower left side of the rib cage. This infection can be very serious for those without a spleen because there is no other way for the infected blood cells to be purified and the spleen serves an important role in immunity.

Many of the symptoms of babesiosis occur because of oxygen deprivation at a cellular level. For example, the low level of oxygen can create anxiety, as if you were holding your breath under water. Once the oxygen starts to run out, you start to feel increased anxiety, prompting you to break through the surface of water for air. Babesiosis patients are usually very oxygen depleted, making them bedbound. Just doing the dishes is exhausting. They will be winded from taking a shower, requiring a nap afterward. Or they may be too tired to shower, which leads to poor self-care and hygiene, purely from lack of energy.

In 2018, the U.S. Food and Drug Administration approved testing of blood, organ, and tissue donations nationwide for *B. microti* using the Imugen Arrayed Fluorescent Immunoassay (AFIA) and Nucleic Acid Test (NAT) in whole blood samples.[38] This will most certainly reduce the transmission of this blood-borne pathogen in the blood supply, which in many cases goes to those who are already immunocompromised.

Symptoms: Symptoms can vary, depending on the immune system's response. The Centers for Disease Control refer to babesiosis as a self-limiting disease, meaning it will resolve on its own. I don't usually see that happen.

A patient will typically have persistent headaches, debilitating fatigue, fevers, chills, sweats, dizziness, enlarged spleen, elevated eosinophils in tissue (which create swelling and allergic-like reactions), petechial rashes (which look like broken blood vessels in the skin), shortness of breath, easy bruising, bone pain, numbness and tingling, abdominal pain, fibromyalgia, nausea, anemia, blood in the urine, and anxiety/depression. Full-body spasmodic episodes that resemble a seizure, occurring daily or a few times per week, may also be a symptom. Patients experience real difficulty multitasking and become overstimulated in public places.

Treatment options: *Pharmaceutical medications*— atovaquone (Mepron), atovaquone/proguanil (Malarone), artemether/lumefantrine (Coartem), hydroxychloroquine (Plaquenil), quinine (Qualaquin). Intravenous medication is clindamycin. Treatment duration is usually at least 120 days, which is the life expectancy of the red blood cell.

Natural treatments—Artemisia, Coptis, Sida acuta, oregano oil, cryptolepis, neem,[39] *Nyctanthes arbor-tristis* Linn.,[40] *Bupleurum*, dandelion, cleavers, blue flag iris

INFECTION WITH HELMINTHS OR AMOEBAS

A variety of larger parasites find the human body a suitable home. These can go unnoticed for years because of their unpredictable life cycles and the body's ability to adapt to their presence. Helminths are flatworms and roundworms that primarily colonize areas of the intestines, though they are not confined to the intestines. Liver flukes, a type of helminth, can move through the body's organ systems and blood, usually finding a home in the liver-gallbladder area. Several symptoms, including poor liver function, fatigue, and irritable bowel syndrome, may well be due to a parasite. Many of my patients over the years have had a spontaneous release of worms in a bowel movement, which was shocking to the individual, to say the least. Whether the release is triggered by a medication or a dietary change, or for an unknown reason, the patient's overall energy generally improves once the worms have been eliminated.

Amoebas are smaller pathogens that colonize the digestive tract, causing mild to severe digestive problems, including dehydration, relapsing diarrhea, gas/bloating, undigested food in stool, and high levels of mucus or blood in the stool. Once in the body, amoebas can stay there for years, slowly growing and shedding at irregular times. Stool analysis can be helpful, but usually more than one sample is necessary to confirm the presence of amoebas; even that does not always work. Amoebas are most commonly transmitted when humans ingest undercooked meats or water tainted with fecal matter or through human-to-human or animal-to-human contact. They are more commonly encountered with international travel but are present in the U.S. water and food supply as well.

Amebiasis and helminth infections are important to mention because of the stress they place on the body by causing malnourishment, increased symptoms associated with autoimmune diseases, allergic reactions, chronic fatigue, changes in organ function, inflammatory bowel disease, and destruction of the gut microbiome, depending on where the infection takes up residence. Infection by these parasites can be a missed complication in a patient who is unable to tolerate medications and has a history of digestive distress. Also, it's not uncommon to have a release of worms or liver flukes while undergoing treatment for tick-borne disease, which can be very distressing to the patient. Several medications used to treat the cyst form of the Lyme disease bacteria are the same as those used to treat worms and parasitic infections.

Symptoms: Most of the symptoms have to do with digestive function, including inflammation of the gastrointestinal lining as the immune system recognizes something that does not belong. As with any parasite, helminths and amoebas feed off the resources of the host, so the infected patient usually experiences weight loss, diarrhea, constipation, bloating, and/or abdominal pain. They may also have stools with mucus, visible blood, or undigested food. Nutrient deficiencies may occur, such as low iron due to poor absorption. Rashes on the skin that come and go as well as itching of the skin are also signs of digestive tract inflammation.

Treatment options: *Pharmaceutical medications*—Tindamax/Flagyl, Alinia, ivermectin

Natural treatments—black walnut, *Artemisia annua* (wormwood), neem, oregano oil, grapefruit seed extract

In Summary

Evaluation and treatment of coinfections are important for a successful recovery. We have all acquired infections as part of our human experience. The microbial world is a highly diverse realm, and understanding this reduces the chance of developing tunnel vision and focusing on one infection. Between infections that come in with the tick and opportunistic infections already present in your system, your treatment may require a diverse array of medications.

The following chapters will review testing and treatment options to help you advocate for yourself as you move toward recovery.

CHAPTER 4

FINDING THE MOST ACCURATE TESTING

A pervasive belief is that if the lab result for Lyme disease is negative, the person must not be infected; however, this is not necessarily so. If your lab result is positive, you have been exposed to the infection; if your lab result is negative, it does not mean you *don't* have Lyme disease. It's common to experience anxiety and indecisiveness after a negative test, when your primary care provider and the Centers for Disease Control are both saying you don't have Lyme disease and only a small group of practitioners across the country is saying you do. It's very difficult to decide to move forward with treatment when there is so much disagreement in the medical field.

Many people are living with Lyme disease and don't know it. They have pain and fatigue but think this is a normal aspect of daily life. How many times do we see commercials promoting pain relievers on TV that make pain look normal? *Functional Lyme patients* are those who have positive titers and history but who have no symptoms. This is more common than you think, and it is why I suggest being tested for Lyme disease yearly if you live in an endemic area. It's just like getting your cholesterol checked. You may not know you were bitten and may not show strong symptoms. It's important to know if you have been exposed so that if your health changes, you can explore Lyme disease as a potential cause.

Many patients who have symptoms but test negative for Lyme disease decide not to treat because they want proof on paper. As much as doctors and patients would like concrete data, the human body does not always show conclusive signs on lab work. A blood test is a snapshot of one moment in time—a small amount of blood vacuumed into a tube at a particular minute is asked to represent what is going on in the body overall. If you tested the same variables throughout the day, many standard tests would show different outcomes. I was taught in medical school that taking a detailed history tells you about 90 percent of what you need to know to make a possible diagnoses, with labs attempting to confirm a concrete diagnosis. If a patient was bitten by a tick and has not felt well since, the cause is pretty clear. The matter becomes more confusing when the patient has no memory of a tick bite.

Many people are living with Lyme disease and don't know it. They have pain and fatigue but think this is a normal aspect of daily life.

Confirming Lyme Disease: ELISA and the Western Blot

The Centers for Disease Control and Prevention (CDC) mandate that the enzyme-linked immunosorbent assay (ELISA) or the C6 antibody screen be run first. These are screening tests, rather than confirmatory ones, and are supposed to be very sensitive, picking up the slightest hint of rising antibodies due to exposure to *Borrelia burgdorferi*. The idea of running these first is to make testing cost effective and to add more data for a firmer diagnosis of Lyme disease. The Western blot is meant to have high specificity for Lyme disease and is the confirmatory test, run only if the ELISA or C6 ELISA is positive.

Unfortunately, the ELISA is not the sensitive test it's purported to be. I have witnessed many false negatives. The common two-tiered testing only looks at one strain of *Borrelia*, though there are more than forty identified strains across the globe, with several specific to the United States. Specialty labs such as IGeneX have a Western blot that takes a more specific look at multiple strains, to give a more diverse view.

Titers (a measure of the presence and number of antibodies in the blood) for infections will vary based on the person's immune status, the stage of infection, and hormone balance. The ELISA and Western blot look at the immune cells produced by the host rather than at the pathogen itself. This method is referred to as *indirect testing*. If you were to look at a lab report for the Western blot, you would see IgM and IgG immunoglobulins produced by the patient's immune system. These are antibodies, proteins produced as a reaction to an infection. Antibodies are categorized based on an atomic weight classification called *kilodaltons* (kDa), with each being given a specific number such as 41 kDa, 23 kDa, or 39 kDa. The bands on the Western blot test represent proteins present when the body comes into contact with *B. burgdorferi* or with parts of the spirochete. For instance, band 39 kDa is specific to the flagella, or tail, of a Lyme disease spirochete. The presence of band 39 kDa is thus indicative of a current infection.

IgM bands are associated with a new, acute infection, or sub-acute active infection, while IgG bands are associated with more long-term, active chronic infections or with antibodies that persist after the infection is resolved. The CDC considers an IgM test positive if two out of three bands are positive; the three bands are 23 kDa, 39 kDa, and 41 kDa. At one time, more bands were required for positive confirmation of an IgM test; the number was slimmed down to just three bands several years ago. For a positive result to be acknowledged for IgG, five bands must be positive out of a possible ten.

As I noted earlier, the Western blot run through conventional labs such as LabCorp or Quest Diagnostics is the confirming test most frequently used. This is partly due to patient preference regarding cost, based on what most insurance will cover. Some patients seek me out specifically to run tests at specialty labs such as IGeneX because they have conducted their own research online and their doctor refuses to run the tests. Many in the medical community believe that the Western blot run at IGeneX labs all come back positive, so the lab must be useless. Many patients have reported that their medical practitioners refuse to even look at their results, saying immediately that the report is inaccurate. After using IGeneX for more than a decade, I can say from experience that this is not true. Many tests return with a negative result, showing no exposure to infection.

When a pregnant woman who has Lyme disease gives birth, the Western blot can be run on the newborn's cord blood. Cord blood is extracted at the time of birth, requiring that a kit be ordered ahead of time, signed off on by the ordering doctor, and taken to the hospital before the date of delivery. This has been really helpful in putting parents' minds at ease about the possibility of transmitting tick-borne infections within the mother to the baby.

I treat empirically based on tick bite history and symptom presentation, informing the patient that we will treat without lab confirmation to see whether there is any change in her health. Remember, there are many strains of *Borrelia*, and every test has its limitations. With the funding constraints for research devoted to this epidemic, we are still at the tip of the iceberg with regard to understanding how to best test for this microbe.

Less Common Tests

While the two-tiered testing of ELISA and the Western blot is most common, other testing methods are available. The polymerase chain reaction (PCR) and culture tests blood, cerebrospinal fluid, biopsied tissue, and fluid pulled from joint spaces. PCR is able to identify and amplify DNA of the microbe within a sample, confirming infection within the body. These testing options are ideal for confirming some infections but are not the most efficient for *B. burgdorferi* because of the PCR's low sensitivity and the difficulty of growing Lyme disease in a culture medium that can be used in a routine clinical setting. It can take anywhere from several weeks to several months to grow spirochetes, due to their replication timing and the fact that they require a very specific environment. The most practical approach is to run blood samples for Western blot initially and to use the PCR and/or culture as second-tier testing.

Another testing option is the dot blot, which is similar to the Western blot but has subtle differences in the specimen type and test procedure. This test requires the patient to take antibiotics and/or natural medications for a period of time to stimulate the release of bacterial debris in the urine. I have not used this test very often in practice, though I know many doctors who use it as their primary testing option. It can be helpful when confirmation is needed for specific treatments or if the patient is not willing or able to give blood. However, cross-reactions with other urinary infections can occur, and other tests should be run to support the diagnosis.

Urine testing using nanoparticles to measure OSP-A proteins created by *B. burgdorferi* is a new option just emerging on the market.

A Balanced Approach to Testing

Lab tests help you understand your internal world and can be life-saving in many cases. It's important to have your lab results reviewed by a doctor who can help you interpret them. In recent years, there has been a lot more freedom surrounding medical testing, with people ordering labs for themselves and

Freak Them Out: Exercise and Natural Medications Can Force Spirochetes into Circulation

BORRELIA **SPIROCHETES HAVE MANY MECHANISMS** in place that allow them to hide from the human immune system, including protection within biofilms, enhanced motility, and dormancy. Before your blood test to check for Lyme disease, try to tease the spirochetes out so the outcome is more apt to be accurate.

Researchers are starting to consider the use of stevia and serrapeptase to enhance PCR testing outcomes because these substances can stimulate the release of more spirochetes in the bloodstream.[1] I suggest taking these supplements one to two weeks before testing to allow the body time to develop any immune reaction.

This not only makes the spirochetes' DNA more bioavailable for PCR testing, but also could improve indirect testing with the Western blot by enhancing IgM and IgG antibodies. Blending both internal biofilm agitators as well as deep tissue massage, different forms of exercise, sauna, or Qigong might also improve the test outcome. This strategy is worth trying if you present with all the symptoms of Lyme disease but have had no confirmation on lab tests.

receiving results before doctors do; but this can lead to confusion. If you start researching on the Internet, you may misinterpret some findings, which leads to fear. This fear can lead you to make assumptions about what you are looking at and possibly cause you to self-diagnose inaccurately.

Approach testing with moderation. Patients often come in asking for "the works," based on their own research or recommendations made by other doctors. When I tell them the cost (thousands of dollars in out-of-pocket expenses) and how many sittings (two or three appointments) it will take to get the amount of blood needed, their list shortens quickly. I can test for everything under the sun, but to what end? In the past, I have agreed to run everything the patient wanted. Thousands of dollars in out-of-pocket expenses later, there was no change to the treatment plan that had been based on the simpler testing approach. Then, there is the other extreme, where patients report that some practitioners are unwilling to run even those tests covered under insurance to screen for tick-borne disease.

Most insurance, I find, will cover tests with mainstream laboratories for tick-borne infections, viral titers, and hormone panels. There are specialty labs that use more sensitive testing for tick-borne infections, inflammation markers, heavy metals, and hormones; and these represent out-of-pocket costs. These tests are run when the situation requires definitive information needed for a more specific diagnosis. I may ask the patient to send out to IGeneX or Galaxy labs to have a more sensitive test performed for *Bartonella* infection if other tests are inconclusive and there is concern about initiating treatment without more information. However, additional testing must always be balanced against the costs; specialty testing can be expensive, and much of it is not covered by insurance.

Routine versus Specialized Testing

I'll discuss first the tests run for the majority of patients; then I'll review those tests run on a case-by-case basis. Most lab results are reevaluated in two- to six-month intervals.

When a patient comes to the clinic concerned about having chronic tick-borne disease, the tests I usually order are Lyme disease Western blot, *Babesia*, *Bartonella*, ehrlichiosis, anaplasmosis, Rocky Mountain spotted fever, Q fever, *Mycoplasma* pneumonia, brucellosis, strep antibodies, CD-57/CD8+, chronic viral infections, *Candida albicans*, hormones, inflammation, complete blood cell count, comprehensive metabolic panel, vitamin status, and autoimmune markers.

Specialized lab tests, which are run on a case-by-case basis, are heavy metal testing; salivary adrenal function testing; stool analysis; nasal culture; test for Ritchie Shoemaker, M.D., biotoxin markers; neurotransmitter testing; tests for food sensitivities; chronic strep infection antibodies; omega fatty acid levels; lipid panel; and Boston Heart Lab.

There are many additional lab tests that might be ordered based on an individual's case, and these are decided by the treating physician. This section provides you with a general understanding of available tests so you can help your doctor in identifying the source of your ill health.

Lab tests are useful in getting objective data, but no test is perfect. As I noted earlier, these tests provide a snapshot of the moment the blood was

The Short Life of the Lyme Disease Vaccine

LYMERIX, THE FIRST AND ONLY LYME DISEASE VACCINE for humans, was approved by the FDA in 1998. It was introduced by GlaxoSmithKline in regions infested with infected ticks and had a very brief life before being withdrawn from the market in 2001. Negative publicity began to swell when a number of patients reported developing Lyme disease–like symptoms after the vaccine was administered. News outlets started to report that the vaccine was harmful.

By the time research was released explaining that the vaccine was not harmful, it had been pulled from the market due to low sales. The vaccine was rejected by the public at a time when Lyme disease was not as big a concern as it is now. The negative reaction to the vaccine was ultimately found to be confined to a subset of the population with the genetic marker HLA-B27, which is associated with autoimmune disease.

Those people who received the vaccine but did not have the genetic marker were tracked for years after being vaccinated and had very low infection rates for Lyme disease. I also believe that many of those vaccinated may have had Lyme disease without knowing it. Being given the vaccine upregulated their immune systems, thus creating a Herxheimer reaction.

A few years after the vaccine was no longer available, the CDC modified the Western blot by removing bands 31 kDa and 34 kDa, which would create a false positive if the person tested had received the vaccination. This is why many people choose to use specialty labs that have this additional information as part of the test. To date, out of the four thousand patients I have treated over the years, I have only met two who had the vaccine. I have always wondered how many people get false negative results now because of this change to the Western blot, which was intended to avoid a very small population of false positives.

taken, and many of the tests will vary in outcome and have different reference ranges provided from different companies for the same test. Also, these ranges change often, based on evolving research. Whereas most tests are automated, some are still being read by humans. The interpretation of the outcome will vary subtly depending on who is doing the reading.

Different doctors also have varying styles, and some prefer to work with certain companies. Doctors also have their own routines and reference ranges they see as optimal. All of these variables can take an objective piece of data and make it quite subjective. This is why lab tests are an amazing set of data, but it's best to be discerning about the outcome.

Common Lab Tests

TESTING IS A SOURCE OF FINANCIAL CONCERN for patients who are trying to get answers without emptying their bank accounts. Lab tests can be a major expense when treating tick-borne disease. The lists below give a rundown of (1) lab tests commonly covered by insurance and (2) specialty tests typically not covered, as they are considered experimental. Many other options for testing exist, but the full complement of tests available is beyond the scope of this book.

Note: Coverage may not be possible for any lab tests, depending on the individual insurance plan and deductible.

ROUTINE LAB TESTS COMMONLY COVERED BY INSURANCE

Coinfection Panel
- *Babesia microti, Babesia duncani, Bartonella henslae,* ehrlichiosis, anaplasmosis, *Mycoplasma* pneumonia, brucellosis, strep antibodies, Rocky Mountain spotted fever

Viral Titer Panel
- Epstein-Barr, parvovirus B19, cytomegalovirus, herpes simplex virus I/II, varicella zoster and human herpesvirus 6
- CD-57/CD8+

Male/Female Hormone Panel
- Estrogens, progesterone, testosterone, dehydroepiandrosterone (DHEA)

Thyroid Hormone Panel
- TSH, free T3, free T4, thyroid antibodies, reverse T3

Inflammation/Autoimmune Panel
- Rheumatoid factor, C-reactive protein, sedimentation rate, CCP antibodies, antinuclear antibodies, and Sjögren's antibodies

Complete Blood Cell Count and Comprehensive Metabolic Panel

Vitamin and Mineral Status
- Vitamin D, vitamin B12, vitamin B6, folate, copper, zinc, magnesium (there is specialty testing for a more comprehensive vitamin analysis)

Candida Antibodies IgM, IgG, IgA

HLA-DR Genetic Panels (Mold-illness, Gluten Intolerance)

Total Immunoglobulin Levels (IgG Subclass, IgM, IgE, IgA)

Gluten Intolerance Testing (Celiac disease)
- Tissue Transglutaminase IgA, IgG (tTG)
- Endomysial Antibodies
- Anti-Gliadin Antibodies

SPECIALTY LAB TESTS
- Adrenal Salivary Index
- Neurotransmitter Panels
- Food Sensitivity Panels
- Heavy Metal Testing
- Stool Analysis
- Genetic Testing
- Nasal Culture
- Small Intestinal Bacterial Overgrowth (SIBO)

The Information Your Body Can Provide

Lab tests can provide objective data that give a more concrete treatment path to follow. The information below provides a deeper understanding of the common tests run and how they measure human health. These tests allow medical providers to individualize care and create a more specific treatment plan, better serving their patients.

CD-57 TEST

The CD-57/CD8+ marker (CD stands for "cluster designation") is used to track a patient's progress through treatment. The CD-57 belongs to a specific immune cell line called a *natural killer cell*. The natural killer cell responds directly to antigens—either toxins or infection—entering the body. Natural killer cells take care of these foreign substances introduced into the body without you even knowing it. They even continuously eliminate precancerous cells, as they recognize these cells are not compatible with maintaining optimal health. Several different CD cells exist, and each has a specific affinity for a type of foreign invader.

The test for CD-57 is not diagnostic for Lyme disease as is the Western blot, but monitoring this marker's levels throughout a patient's treatment process helps evaluate the individual's response to treatment. I use this test to track the activity of these cells, taking the patient's original number and following it like an infant growth chart. This test is repeated every three to six months and used as another piece of data to track a patient's response to treatment. The test can also indicate if a patient is having a relapse.

Published research, primarily by Raphael Stricker, M.D., has shown a correlation between lower CD-57 levels and potential risk of relapse in chronic Lyme disease.[2] Further studies have also shown a strong correlation between an abnormal CD-57, usually decreased, and the several autoimmune diseases.[3] The reference range is 60–360 cells per microliter of blood. Most chronic Lyme disease patients are below 60 cells per microliter of blood. A level lower than 100 is undesirable, and the goal is to have this immune cell living in healthy numbers of around 200–360 in the human body.

It's important, however, to remember that this is simply a marker and not to get attached to it. Over the years, I have seen in my patients a correlation between CD-57 and chronic Lyme disease, with lower numbers also in those with reactivated Epstein-Barr virus and coinfection with *Babesia* species. Try not to become preoccupied with the CD-57 result if the number is less than you were hoping for. For some people, it takes longer for this number to return to normal than it does for others. What matters most is how you feel.

MALE/FEMALE HORMONE PANELS

Hormones play an important role in immune function, support of proper growth and development, and healthy energy levels. When persistent infections exist, glandular function can decrease, there may be poor communication between the brain and glands, and changes in hormone balance can occur in both genders. This seems to happen to people in just about every age category, affecting energy level, libido, sleep cycles, mood, cognition, and healthy biological functions. Nearly all my patients have some form of hormone imbalance. This test can also be used to make sure bioidentical hormone doses are healthy and in balance. Treatment can be easily modified with the support of testing to optimize the dosage for the patient's individual needs.

THYROID HORMONE PANEL

The thyroid is one of the glands of survival, managing the body's metabolism in times of health and when the body is under stress. Tick-borne diseases, dietary sensitivities, and toxins can change the function of the thyroid gland, leading to either overproduction or underproduction of thyroid hormones. It's common for the immune system to attack the thyroid, creating antibodies that heighten or lower the function of the thyroid. This can happen because of genetic predisposition, infections, toxins, or food intolerances such as celiac disease.

To get an overall view of thyroid health, I recommend testing the thyroid hormones T3 and T4 as well as the thyroid antibodies. To test the health of the thyroid, physicians usually run a test that checks the levels of thyroid-stimulating hormone (TSH). This is the hormone the brain secretes to communicate with the thyroid, allowing it to maintain proper function. Testing all these parameters—T3, T4, antibodies, and TSH—is necessary to assess hormone function and devise the most effective treatment, if needed.

Treatment of imbalance is usually herbal medication or bioidentical hormone replacement therapy. Symptoms of low-functioning thyroid are weight gain, constipation, and changes in hair, skin, and nails. Elevated blood pressure or low blood pressure can also be present. In my practice, I see more low-functioning thyroid than hyperfunctioning thyroid. Reduced thyroid function is due to autoimmune attack of the thyroid or low hormone output due to the gland being overwhelmed by prolonged illness in the body.

Some patients have had the thyroid removed or the gland killed with radioactive iodine to stop overproduction of thyroid hormones. Those without thyroid function are treated as hypothyroid patients and prescribed thyroid medication. If a problem with the thyroid exists, there is almost

Lyme disease, because it can move into body spaces such as joint capsules, muscles, organs, and tissue, can be a catalyst for developing an autoimmune disease.

certainly a problem with its partner, the adrenal glands. Iodine blood levels may be checked if low-functioning thyroid occurs without signs of autoantibody attack. Iodine is a nutrient requirement for proper thyroid function.

INFLAMMATION/AUTOIMMUNE PANEL

The autoimmune panel expands my differential diagnosis (the process of differentiating between conditions that share similar symptoms) to rule out the presence of lupus, Sjögren's syndrome, rheumatoid arthritis, juvenile rheumatoid arthritis, mixed connective tissue diseases, and others. Lyme disease, because it can move into body spaces such as joint capsules, muscles, organs, and tissue, can be a catalyst for developing an autoimmune disease. Both can happen at the same time. A patient may require care from a rheumatologist to provide necessary medications to find relief of symptoms. I always encourage patients to seek second opinions and work with other specialists as needed.

An additional test that is important for those who experience persistent joint pain despite treatment for Lyme disease detects the presence of the human leukocyte antigen B27 (HLA-B27) marker on white blood cells. This specific HLA on your white blood cells can cause your immune system to attack itself under certain stressful conditions. Immune cells with this particular marker are implicated in attacking connective tissue in the body, and these cells have been linked to reactive arthritis when triggered by an event such as a microbe entering the body. Those who have this marker also have a higher likelihood of developing ankylosing spondylitis, which causes inflammation of the bones in the spine.

COMPLETE BLOOD CELL (CBC) COUNT AND COMPREHENSIVE METABOLIC PANEL

These are standard blood tests used by every medical practice in the world. This panel gives a general overview of the health of the immune system, the kidneys, and the liver, as well as electrolyte levels. The tests provide useful information for monitoring the body throughout the treatment process for Lyme disease to make sure no unwanted side effects from medications occur and that there is no trauma to the organs for other reasons. The most common abnormalities I see are slightly elevated liver enzymes and anemia. Among my patients, it is rare for these tests to come back showing severe complications. The CBC and metabolic panel are always helpful for a patient who is uncomfortable about the use of antibiotic or other medications—seeing on paper that their health is not adversely affected by the treatment means they have one less concern.

VITAMIN AND MINERAL STATUS REPORT

Vitamin and mineral levels commonly tested are iron (including ferritin levels), vitamin D, B12, folate, B6, zinc, magnesium, and copper. These can all be depleted with long-term illness, poor digestive health, and long-term use of antacids (which most patients have been prescribed prior to presenting to the clinic). Nutrient deficiency can contribute to adrenal fatigue, anxiety, depression, muscle cramps, cardiovascular instability, enhanced metabolic risk factors, and poor concentration.

Vitamin and mineral levels are easily tested through conventional labs such as LabCorp or Quest Diagnostics, which makes insurance coverage more likely; but micronutrient testing available from companies such as SpectraCell Laboratories offers a more in-depth look at your current vitamin status and immune function. Micronutrient panels such as those offered by SpectraCell are typically not covered by insurance. They are valuable in providing a snapshot of your current vitamin, amino acid, and mineral status but do represent an out-of-pocket expense. Looking at nutrient deficiencies can help you give your body exactly what you need for optimal health.

Vitamin D is discussed in further detail in chapter 8. This essential vitamin is typically low in most of my patients unless they are already supplementing it on their own. The optimal level for this vitamin and hormone is 60–70 ng/ml, whereas most Lyme disease patients have very low levels, below 30 ng/ml.

TEST FOR *CANDIDA* ANTIBODIES

Whether or not a patient reports symptoms associated with yeast overgrowth, such as skin rashes, nail bed infections, sugar cravings, oral lesions, digestive complaints, or vaginal irritation with discharge, I test routinely for Candida antibodies. If the body is creating antibodies against Candida albicans, immunity can be reduced and inflammation increased. This can make treatment more difficult if Candida is not addressed with proper dietary changes and antifungal medications. Levels of Candida antibodies are monitored routinely throughout treatment when antimicrobials are used due to the possibility of yeast overgrowth as a byproduct of treatment. The microbiome requires utmost support with prebiotics, probiotics, and significantly reduced sugar consumption during the treatment process to avoid overgrowth of unwanted guests such as nonbeneficial yeast. One way to counter unwanted microbes is with the therapeutic use of the beneficial yeast culture Saccharomyces boulardii.

HLA-DR GENETIC PANEL

The HLA-DR genetic panel requires a decoder, known as the Rosetta Stone, developed by Dr. Shoemaker. The test looks at different codes that represent gene pathways that enhance a person's sensitivities to mold biotoxin. I will not go into great depth about the tests and will instead refer you to www.survivingmold.com, which provides resources for those suffering ill effects from mold exposure.

The lab values from this test show the level of inflammation and hormone imbalance in the body, a possible result of the internal environment accumulating too many toxins from microbes. Many patients commonly live or work in environments that harbor toxic mold due to water damage. This can compound the symptoms of chronic Lyme disease, making it more difficult for the person to function. Dr. Shoemaker's approach addresses the inflammatory stress that comes from chronic Lyme disease, as well as from mold toxins and resistant infections of the sinus cavity.

Those who are positive for the genetic markers on this test have a reduced capacity to clear the mold toxins from the body; these toxins can create brain fog, fatigue, body pain, neurological dysfunction, nausea, headaches, visual disturbances, rashes, breathing difficulty, and mood changes.

Treatment is centered on releasing the toxins through specific medications, making changes in the environment to improve air quality, and enhancing the immune system. Symptoms of toxic mold exposure are similar to those commonly seen in chronic Lyme disease. In fact, there is a genetic pattern tested within the HLA-DR panel for individuals who have reduced capacity to clear the toxins created by *Borrelia burgdorferi*. Based on the outcome of the genetic testing, the following tests may be done as a further study of body burden:

- Melanocyte-stimulating hormone, C4a, C3a, TGFβ-1, VEGF, anti-cardiolipins, antidiuretic hormones, matrix metallopeptidase 9 (MMP-9), and leptin. These are all components that, when put together, can raise the stress on the system from biotoxin overload. Seek out a medical practitioner familiar with Dr. Shoemaker's approach to get the best interpretation of these tests.
- Visual Contrast Sensitivity APTitude Test: This test is available at www.survivingmold.com. I frequently suggest that patients conduct this test; it is reasonably priced and very helpful in determining biotoxin body burden and the impact of biotoxins on the nervous system. The result can be tracked over time to assess treatment progress.

For further information on mold toxins, testing, and treatment, I recommend *Surviving Mold* by Dr. Ritchie Shoemaker.

IMMUNOGLOBULIN LEVELS

Immunoglobulins are also known as antibodies, which are created by plasma cells. Looking for antibodies is the most common method to confirm infections in the body, including Lyme disease (with the Western blot). Antibodies can be categorized into classes IgA, IgD, IgE, IgG, and IgM. The primary immunoglobulins tested are IgA, IgE, IgM, and IgG. Each has a specific purpose in the body. IgE is most present at times of immediate allergic reaction, such as a person's allergic response to peanuts or bee stings. In the context of Lyme disease treatment, the focus is primarily on IgM and IgG. IgM immunoglobulin is usually the first marker to show in a new infection. With Lyme disease, IgM can keep upregulating over and over like a brand-new infection as the spirochetes reproduce, triggering the immune system to react as if it's seeing the infection for the first time.

IgG subclass testing is an important panel to perform routinely. The most prolific antibody that shows up in later-stage infection, IgG maintains human immunity throughout the whole body from birth. Lyme disease patients can have a deficiency in this immunoglobulin, which makes it difficult for the body to mount an appropriate response to clear the infection.

Low IgG also correlates with inflammatory conditions that cause nerve damage, such as Guillain-Barré and chronic inflammatory demyelinating polyneuropathy (CIDP); this damage can be confirmed with a biopsy of tissue taken from the affected area.

The treatment for the condition is called *intravenous immunoglobulin therapy* (IVIg) and involves replacing the immunoglobulin IgG. It's currently not approved for use with Lyme disease, but clinically there is a correlation between those with rapidly progressive neurological decline and low IgG levels. If this level is low in a Lyme disease patient, the next step is to see a neurologist or immunologist to evaluate for IVIg treatment. It takes hundreds of donors to yield just one dose, and the price per dose is several thousand dollars. This treatment is very difficult to get covered by insurance, but I have seen it really improve a patient's quality of life and ability to fight infections.

GLUTEN INTOLERANCE TESTING

This test is done to rule out celiac disease or gluten intolerance. Unfortunately, if a person had a slight intolerance to gluten before contracting Lyme disease, that intolerance will magnify in a majority of patients. Stress on the immune system can prompt an improper immune response to foods. With gluten sensitivity or celiac disease, an overabundance of autoimmune antibodies created in response to gluten exposure leads to inflammation in the body, negatively impacting cognition, skin, respiratory health, thyroid balance, and energy levels; the condition creates body pain as well. Gluten proteins can also wear away the lining of the gut, making it difficult to absorb proper nutrition.

Gluten intolerance is a gray area and may not show up positive on lab results, as celiac disease does. Most Lyme disease patients should reduce or eliminate gluten as part of their treatment process, to reduce inflammation in the body. This will also significantly reduce the intake of sugar, which has its own health implications. Many patients on gluten-free diets show improvements in symptoms that have been present most of their lives, such as digestive imbalance, postnasal drip, unwanted weight, and acne.

This is one of those tests that, if positive, means you really need to remove gluten, but if negative, it is still worth trying a 30-day restriction period to see whether it makes a difference in your health. However, most people want to see the need on paper before ditching one of their favorite food categories. The most common way to determine a diagnosis of celiac disease is through tests for tissue transglutaminase, endomysial antibodies, and gliadin antibodies.

Specialty Testing

Each medical specialty has its own way of using laboratory medicine to diagnose illness. There are tests that are standard across all specialties, and then there are those tests that look in greater depth at more specific data. In the naturopathic medical community, we use lab tests to look at detox pathways, gauge food intolerance, assess toxic burden in the body caused by heavy metals, evaluate hormones, and analyze stool analysis to expand on possible causes for digestive distress. Whether you are seeing a naturopathic doctor for Lyme disease or for another reason, these common tests are used in the naturopathic medical community to craft an individualized treatment plan. Because many of these tests are not embraced by the allopathic medical community, they may not be covered by insurance. The good news is that many of the tests are reasonably priced for most patients.

ADRENAL SALIVARY INDEX
The adrenal glands sit atop the kidneys and play several roles in the body, including balancing blood sugar, helping the body adapt to stress, maintaining a proper sleep schedule, and regulating the immune system. When the adrenal glands are not functioning properly, quality of life can be compromised. The preferred test measures hormone levels in saliva, the best method for measuring free, active levels (adrenal hormones are either inactive—bound to a protein—or active—freely roaming).

One of the most important components of the test is the graph of cortisol output, which shows the trend of this hormone from early morning to before bed. This requires four collections of saliva through the day at specific intervals. Cortisol is expressed as a response to adrenaline output; it smooths out physical, mental, and emotional responses to stress and helps in recovery. Over time, if adrenaline production is constantly being stimulated by trauma, anxiety, unusual physical demands, or pain, energy reserves will decrease, leading to poor recovery and physical health.

Cortisol is at its peak in the morning, to get you out of bed, and then it gradually reduces throughout the day so you are ready for bed in the late evening. Many Lyme disease patients have cortisol levels that are either flat or have the curves reversed, with the lowest levels produced in the morning hours and higher levels at night. This creates an altered sleep schedule, so you are up late at night and sleep later in the day.

NEUROTRANSMITTER PANELS

Neurotransmitter panels are urinary and salivary hormone panels conducted to assess the levels of histamine, serotonin, norepinephrine, dopamine, gamma-aminobutyric acid (GABA), PEA, epinephrine, and glutamate. Proper balance of these hormones promotes quality sleep, concentration, balanced mood, and healthy appetite, all of which are altered when the body has chronic active infections.

If testing shows that neurohormones are out of balance, natural medications in the form of botanicals and amino acids can work more effectively, in many cases, than prescription medications. In other cases, prescription medications may be required but natural medications may help reduce the amount needed.

FOOD SENSITIVITY PANELS

The increase in genetically modified foods, hormones given to poultry and livestock, and pesticides used on produce has certainly changed the human body's relationship with food. With most common foods, the immune system should not mount a response that causes chronic infection. If a triggering food is identified and removed from the diet, dramatic improvements in chronic health complaints can take place quickly. Food intolerance testing can be very helpful in providing a clear guide to the foods that trigger your body. The most common food triggers positive on patient lab results are gluten/gliadin-containing grains, bovine dairy, eggs, baker's yeast, and sugarcane. The tests are intuitive to read and look at more than one hundred different foods.

Typically, allergists test by skin scraping or pinprick testing, where the allergen is introduced into deeper layers of the skin. Then the skin is observed for a reaction of redness, swelling, or hives. This method tests a common immunoglobulin, IgE, which is primarily responsible for the anaphylactic response. I don't want to understate the importance of testing for IgE, which is responsible for acute reactions such as those experienced by people with severe peanut allergies; knowing about the allergy could mean life or death. Sensitivities that cause more chronic conditions such as asthma, eczema, digestive issues, fatigue, brain fog, and postnasal drip are due to elevated IgG immunoglobulins rather than IgE. Thus, these standard skin tests may not reveal a chronic food sensitivity. IgG is the most copious immunoglobulin in the body and is there to fight invaders. With certain immune dysfunction, the immunoglobulin starts to perceive foods as invaders.

HEAVY METAL TESTING

With the assistance of the provoking agents dimercaptosuccinic acid (DMSA), ethylenediaminetetraacetic acid (EDTA), 2,3-dimercapto-1-propanesulfonic acid (DMPS), or glutathione (chelating agents), the body can release metals that have been retained in tissues for years. After oral ingestion or intravenous dosing of the chelating agent, urine is collected for eight to twenty-four hours. The medication binds the metals, pulling them from tissues; the metals are then quickly eliminated by the body. Metals commonly tested are mercury, arsenic, lead, nickel, uranium, cadmium, aluminum, and other by-products of industry that are released into water, leach into food, and are airborne on dust particles.

There is a correlation between heavy metals retained in the body and reduced energy, which is needed to fully recover from chronic infections. However, I typically focus on the infection first because the microbes can replicate and migrate through the body. Metals are stored in tissue, making them less reactive than the infections floating freely in the blood. Blood tests run by conventional labs show more recent exposure to metals. Bioaccumulation over time requires a stimulant to release the metals in the body; for the provocation testing, you will likely have to seek out a complementary and alternative practitioner.

I can't stress enough the importance of having this process managed by a doctor trained in chelation therapy. You need to be monitored for healthy liver and kidney function as well as for proper nutrient status. Chelation will remove the minerals you do want as well as the metals you don't. Do not attempt to self-treat with DMSA or EDTA ordered online, as you could cause yourself harm. Chelation medications are usually very well tolerated, and a trained practitioner will do a proper screening to determine whether you are a healthy candidate for chelation. Herbs and amino acids can support gentle metal release, and these are fine to self-prescribe; they include chlorella, parsley, zeolites, sodium alginate, modified citrus pectin, N-acetyl-cysteine, vitamin C, glutathione, sauna, and gentle fasts.

STOOL ANALYSIS

This is probably one of the most humbling tests for patients to complete, as it involves collecting a stool specimen. It's less invasive than colonoscopy as an initial screen of bowel health. Stool analysis testing can be important in identifying inflammation in the bowels, bacterial imbalance, fungal overgrowth, decreased pancreatic function, malabsorption, and parasitic infections. Samples are usually taken in two- to three-day intervals to try to capture certain parasites that shed at random times.

Stool analysis is recommended when the patient has intense abdominal pain with diarrhea, chronic constipation, blood in stool, copious mucus in stool, intense odor beyond the usual, and/or rapid weight loss. Specialty labs (DiagnosTechs, Genova Labs) provide a more comprehensive analysis, but tests are typically not covered by insurance.

We are learning more about the power of our choices— through proper nutrition, toxin reduction, and positive changes in our mental-emotional life— to de-emphasize genes that are not in our favor.

GENETIC TESTING

We all want to understand ourselves in a deeper way. Genetic testing with companies such as AncestryDNA and 23andMe, as well as nutrigenomic testing, in which genetic and individualized nutrition analysis meet, give us inside information so we can better understand our lineage and improve our self-care. Genetic testing can show how you process medications, how to be more proactive about health issues that run in your family, how you best detoxify, your optimal nutrition, and what types of medications can be most effective for you. There is usually a two-tiered approach to genetic testing, with one lab providing codes in alphanumeric form. These results then need to be sent to a separate company such as Genetic Genie, Xcode Life, or Strate-Gene that, for a fee, interprets the results.

Knowledge without proper context can be a hindrance rather than a help. Sometimes, patients come to me practically in tears because of a genetic test they believe will determine their story. I caution patients to be careful about believing that they are doomed by their genes. The intended outcome of genetic testing is to understand possibilities, which is all they are.

The good news is that there is a field called *epigenetics* that studies the body's ability to turn genes on and off without changing the genetic code. The human genome may be an iron-clad code, but that does not mean we are doomed. We are learning more about the power of our choices—through proper nutrition, toxin reduction, and positive changes in our mental-emotional life—to de-emphasize genes that are not in our favor. We have the power to improve our health by seeing ourselves as healthy, improving self-care, and healing our emotional wounds to improve the story written in our genetic code.

NASAL CULTURE

Nasal culture is helpful in identifying chronic infection of the sinuses, especially MARCoNS (multiple antibiotic resistant coagulase negative staph) infection high up in the nasal passages. Chronic sinus infections such as MARCoNS can lower immunity, and the presence of this and other infections can increase inflammation in the body, increase biofilm production, lower white blood cell counts, and create chronic fatigue. Nasal culture is important to do if there are symptoms of recurrent sinus infections, persistent runny nose, or known mold exposure, and for those with a history of chronic Lyme disease.

This simple test involves swabbing the nasal passages to collect a sample and sending it to the lab to see what grows based on your flora. The test typically used in my office is through the laboratory Microbiology DX, and it's relatively inexpensive given the data it provides. If a pathogen grows in culture, this lab will do a sensitivity test, which shows the most effective antibiotics to treat the infection. A positive test can also be matched with the biotoxin markers HLA-DR to get a more well-rounded picture of the body's overload of biotoxins, based on the protocol created by Dr. Shoemaker to identify the impact of MARCoNS on the system. These can also be revisited to check patient recovery posttreatment.

SMALL INTESTINAL BACTERIAL OVERGROWTH (SIBO) HYDROGEN BREATH TEST

SIBO is the presence of higher levels of bacteria normally found in the colon, which may migrate to the small bowel. This is another disease that was characterized as psychosomatic until the scientific community gained a greater understanding of the biodiversity and function of the microbiome.

The digestive tract houses trillions upon trillions of microbes that are viral, bacterial, and fungal and that create a protective barrier as well as educate the immune system. However, a particular order must be maintained because microbes that are beneficial in one area quickly become pathogenic in another area of the gut. An individual's microbiota is like a unique fingerprint, with certain strains of microbes living in specific areas of the small or large intestine. When microbes migrate they cause a change in population, which can irritate the digestive tract, triggering irritable bowel symptoms, body pain, motility issues, leaky gut, fatigue, weight changes, and rashes on the skin. This condition seems to be found more in women and in those who are taking acid-blocking medications, have a history of irritable bowel syndrome, or a history of narcotic use.[4]

The gold standard for confirming a diagnosis of SIBO involves extracting a bacterial sample from the jejunum of the small intestine, but this is cost prohibitive and is also invasive. The most commonly ordered test is the hydrogen breath test; for this test, breath samples are collected every twenty minutes over the course of two to three hours, and both hydrogen and methane gases are tested. The output is measured to determine whether there is an overpopulation of certain methane-producing bacteria. To get accurate results, the patient must follow specific instructions to avoid certain foods and medications several weeks before the test is administered. Treatment is either with antibiotics such as Xifaxan or with antimicrobial herbal protocols, many of which are commonly used with tick-borne infection.

In Summary

We all like to see evidence on paper that validates and confirms the cause of our discomfort. As much as you may want answers, take it step by step when ordering lab tests, to mitigate out-of-pocket expenses. Don't get discouraged if lab results don't always reflect what you want or how you feel. Don't view tests as the be-all and end-all in defining your health. Instead, look at them as valuable tools to help in diagnosis and treatment.

PART

2

FINDING
RELIEF

CHAPTER 5

STEPPING INTO YOUR POWER: SELF-ADVOCACY AND TREATMENT

No matter their age or background, Lyme disease patients have in common their struggle to find a doctor who will treat them appropriately as well as their stories of pushing through a system in which they always seem to be chasing other diagnoses. There is a learning curve in having a controversial disease. You may never have experienced discrimination before, but you might in this situation—and it will require that you grow a thicker skin. Other people do not have to agree with the diagnosis of Lyme disease, but they need to treat you with compassion and respect. We know boundaries are being crossed when we start to avoid interactions with others or feel constricted inside when in someone's presence. If you can't tell your practitioner you are concerned about Lyme disease without him shooting you down or talking to you disrespectfully, it's time to find another practitioner.

The ideal attitude from a health care provider who is unconvinced of a Lyme disease diagnosis should be: "I may not agree with the diagnosis, but I support your choice. Keep me updated." Often, the conversation is much more hostile, and I hear of doctors who have gotten up and walked out when a patient initiates a conversation about Lyme disease. I mention this not because I want to throw other doctors under the bus but because the dismissive attitude of many in the medical community has become a significant problem for patients seeking diagnosis and treatment.

We all deserve to be respected, to be heard, and to feel safe when we enter into a professional relationship with a physician. This partnership between doctor and patient should be an open dialogue in which the goal is to find the best solution for the patient. Being a Lyme-literate doctor demands a particular skill set, and it's important that the doctor understand the process of the disease so she can navigate challenges safely on behalf of the patient, as the treatment can become difficult for many. It is also critical that the practitioner understand the politics surrounding Lyme disease and the daily challenges a Lyme disease patient faces so she can support the patient.

When you test with a specialist who is Lyme literate, you are working with someone who has experience following chronic tick-borne disease patients over time and who understands the unique aspects of the recovery process. Such specialists realize the importance of running a comprehensive panel of tests to assess your health status and understand how to interpret lab results properly.

Many primary care providers are very much in favor of referring patients to specialists such as me and are supportive of patients working with a doctor who has more experience treating the condition. A good working relationship between practitioners makes recovery more successful for patients and their families.

Too often, however, I have to give emotional support and do damage control after patients have difficult interactions with other practitioners. These are doctors who, unfortunately, judge a patient's condition inaccurately, quoting the Centers for Disease Control's current Lyme Disease Treatment Guidelines. Unfortunately, these providers do not always do this in a kind way, and patients may require emotional support to understand what took place with a doctor they have trusted for years.

A great deal of misinformation and miscommunication could be avoided if medical professionals who resist the idea of chronic Lyme disease would soften their approach with patients. This does not mean they have to agree with a diagnosis of chronic Lyme disease, but they should voice their opinions in a respectful way and be open to the patient's concerns.

The Best of Both Worlds: A Balanced Approach to Care

Working with a provider who can balance the use of natural medicine with conventional medications is essential. A practitioner who is steeped in natural medications only, such as a skilled herbalist or one with a certificate in homeopathy, will be knowledgeable in the use of these therapeutics but won't have the necessary training in pharmacology. Medical doctors who have not completed special training in natural medicine or functional medicine will only feel comfortable with prescription medications. Tick-borne infections require both.

Natural medicine can make the difference in whether a patient makes it through the treatment.

Natural medicine can make the difference in whether a patient makes it through the treatment because these natural approaches can help keep gut health safe and avoid serious infections such as *Clostridium difficile*, which occur when there is inadequate flora in the gastrointestinal tract. There are also many natural ways to promote healthy detoxification, immune support, and hormone support throughout the process, reducing treatment time and side effects. Conventional medications are helpful for many acute and chronic conditions; however, there is always room to balance the care with natural medicine and other alternative healing modalities that improve quality of life.

Often, patients treat with conventional medical doctors who have no training or confidence in the use of natural medicine. These doctors may instruct patients not to take natural medicines, including probiotics, because they hold a belief, based on their education, that natural medicine is not useful. On the flip side, natural medicine practitioners can be convinced that conventional medications are dangerous, and they can be just as extreme regarding use of prescription medications.

Patients over the years have reported feeling confused about whom to listen to. What is the truth? It's important to be discerning in the practitioners you see and to find a balanced approach to your care. The ideal is a provider who can pull from different modalities with an open mind.

Tick-borne disease tends to bring on controversy and debate, fueling division when the solution is unity. We need all hands on deck to treat what is already an epidemic and to prepare for what is to come with this emerging infection. Awareness of chronic Lyme disease will hit a tipping point where we can no longer argue over its existence and will have no choice except to face it head-on. There will no longer be time to indulge in debate.

This book represents my own experience, but there are many different styles and protocols out there. My training started with the International Lyme and Associated Diseases Society (ILADS) practitioners, but my teachers are the thousands of patients I have worked with over the years. The best advice I can give is stay on the middle path. Pull from all modalities that feel good to you. A cornucopia of options exists, including pharmaceuticals, natural medications, stem cell treatments, dietary changes, energy-healing modalities, and physical medicine.

You may be compelled to try treatments that in the past you would have thought of as wacky. The thought of reading a book by a naturopathic doctor might never have entered your mind six months ago. Yet you are doing it because you want to get well as soon as you can. This desire may propel you to finally quit smoking, make healthy dietary changes, work on your past traumas, change behaviors that have held you back, or alter your life course in a way that you could never have imagined otherwise. So, you embrace the wacky in the hope of returning to normalcy. Remember, though, that many treatments that are now common practice were at one time laughed at.

Always question whether a path feels right for you. Question what is being offered, the motivation of the practitioner, and what that practitioner is charging. Is the practitioner promising what you want to hear, though it may not be an appropriate guarantee? Be judicious. If the practitioner promises a cure or tells you you're a quick fix then asks for a big up-front payment, be wary. If, on the other hand, you feel that a particular practice is where you belong for your recovery, follow your instinct. Choosing a treatment solely out of fear or bouncing from doctor to doctor trying to find a quick fix will exhaust both you and your wallet.

Finding the Ideal Medication Regimen

The most common antibiotic prescribed for tick-borne disease in people over the age of ten is doxycycline (for children under eleven and pregnant women, penicillin or cephalosporin are the antibiotics of choice). Minocycline is the next-generation drug after doxycycline. I prefer to prescribe minocycline because it's easier on the patient's digestive system and has reduced sun sensitivity, a common problem with doxycycline. Minocycline can create pressure in the head, which usually subsides. Most patients can tolerate the full dose, but it can also be started at a low dose and increased gradually to avoid this side effect. Minocycline crosses into the brain, which is preferable in a drug used to treat an infection that can migrate into the brain.

As we saw earlier, the spirochetes change form, and as this happens a different medication is required to have an impact on the microbe. The spiral form is most susceptible to the tetracycline family of medications, while the L-form is more treatable with cephalosporins and penicillins. The cyst form requires antiprotozoal medications, such as Flagyl, Tindamax, or Alinia, to break through the cell wall and treat the infection. This is why patients working with a Lyme-literate doctor often take more than one antibiotic at a time. Coinfections, discussed in chapter 3, may also require that another specific medication be coadministered. Such complex medical scenarios mean that the conventional medicine protocols currently recommended may not be long enough or diverse enough to overcome the infection.

There are a lot of divergent opinions on the use of antibiotics. Many doctors are emphatically in favor of their use, while others insist that antibiotics will just make matters worse by driving the infection deeper into tissues and creating more resistant strains. One to two weeks of medication might be enough for some people, while others require longer treatment time. Short-course antibiotics might reduce symptoms and give the false impression the infection has cleared, only to resurface weeks or months later. It's important to treat each case individually, treating until symptoms are resolved and then continuing for an additional period of time to avoid relapse.

It's important to weigh the risks and benefits of antibiotic use. Through years of clinical experience with long-term antibiotics, I have seen these medications work to help resolve infections or return quality of life to people who have struggled with Lyme disease. Antibiotics have changed the course of many patients' lives, so I use them when it's appropriate. Do they work in every situation? No. Nothing works all the time. The best treatment protocol is designed around individual needs. It's also important, when treating with antibiotics, to support the body with probiotics, prebiotics, and herbal and nutrient support (discussed in chapter 7) to avoid side effects and long-term complications.

A common erroneous assumption by the conventional medical community is that the use of antibiotics for Lyme disease is not effective beyond fourteen to twenty-eight days. Debate about treatment duration and persistence of infection forms the chief controversy surrounding Lyme disease. Many doctors have lost their good standing in the medical community and have had their licenses suspended or been put under a great deal of scrutiny for treating outside the confines of the Infectious Diseases Society of America (IDSA) guidelines outlined in the sidebar "What We Resist, Persists" in this chapter. Research on Lyme disease treatment has been extremely biased in support of the guidelines, with few resources devoted to studying outcomes with long-term antibiotics.

Research conducted in opposition to the IDSA guidelines has focused on proving that Lyme disease persists in the body beyond the conventional treatment time in a significant number of patients. The IDSA support for those suffering from post-treatment Lyme disease syndrome (PTLDS) are lacking in criteria for addressing persistent body pain, fatigue, and neurological symptoms. An article published in the *International Journal of Infectious Disease* titled "Development of a Foundation for a Case Definition of Post-treatment Lyme Disease Syndrome" says, "the stated criteria leave much open to interpretation. With no standardized approach to capturing the symptoms and functional impact, clinicians and researchers are left to decide on their own. It is unknown how often or in what manner these criteria are applied."[1]

In one study, published in 2017 in *PLoS One*, researchers inoculated ten monkeys using ticks infected with *Borrelia burgdorferi*. One out of ten of these monkeys developed a confirmed bull's-eye rash, which indicates the significant variability of rash presentation. This reflects humans' inconsistent presentation of the bull's-eye rash. Researchers reported that the monkey with the rash did not show positive antibodies upon testing, as the others did, which was an interesting finding. Other forms of testing, including tissue samples, showed that the monkey with the rash did indeed have a confirmed exposure. Their theory was that the spirochetes might have stayed in the skin for a longer period of time, delaying the overall antibody response.

Testing was unable to show consistency with antibody response in antibiotic-treated monkeys versus untreated monkeys. The treated monkeys were given a twenty-eight-day course of doxycycline sixteen weeks after inoculation.[2] All the monkeys were tracked for months afterward to check antibody variability, and persistent *B. burgdorferi* was found in both cohorts— the five treated with an antibiotic and the five left untreated.

This type of research is essential because there is so much certainty in the current medical model that spirochetes do not and cannot persist after medication has been administered. This is a common belief communicated by medical professionals based on the constructs of the IDSA criteria. Testing and the presence of a rash are used as criteria for administering treatment. Yet how can these be the only criteria when there is so much variability in host immunity, coinfections, bite location, genetic predisposition, and the variability of immunoglobulins used to confirm presence? Lyme disease persists; this is the core truth.

If you accept that Lyme disease persists, it's clear that continued treatment of some sort would be more advantageous than throwing our hands in the air and saying there is nothing else that can be done. Remember, many Lyme disease patients, particularly those who live in an endemic area, have accumulated exposure to tick-borne infections over time. Seeing a patient with persistent symptoms and not using available therapies to treat an infection does not make sense, considering the risk-to-benefit of developing chronic illness in the future. This failure to treat concerns not only Lyme disease but also other infections such as babesiosis, anaplasmosis, bartonellosis, and

Rocky Mountain spotted fever, which can also persist; all are placed under the same umbrella as Lyme disease, even though they might involve a very different morphological experience in the body and could require antibiotics different from those that would be prescribed for Lyme disease.

I have not personally seen antibiotics create severe irreversible immune dysfunction or issues with drug resistance, which is frequently quoted as a reason to refrain from treating with antibiotics. I have treated more than four thousand patients with tick-borne disease, and I can say that treatment—whether it is with antibiotics, natural medicine, or an integrative medicine approach—overwhelmingly improves a patient's health status as the infections/toxins are cleared and the immune system becomes able to fully recover. Treatment for tick-borne infection is not a one-size-fits-all process, and each patient's journey is different.

A Complementary and Alternative Medicine Approach

This is an interesting time for Lyme disease: There is a great deal of denial and many polarized views regarding the disease in mainstream medicine, and the gap is being filled by complementary and alternative medicine (CAM), which is bringing forward promising new treatments. These innovative therapies include hyperthermia treatments, low-dose immunotherapy, healing with oxygen, nutraceuticals, intravenous medical protocols with ultraviolet light, intravenous nutrient therapies, stem cell therapies, botanical/essential oils as antimicrobials, energy medicine, and magnetic therapies. We will discuss many of these treatments further in upcoming chapters.

Most medical trade shows and conventions for tick-borne disease focus on CAM therapies, and vendors fill the halls so that doctors can learn all that natural medicine has to offer. The train is rolling, and more practitioners are jumping on board because the complementary medicine approach works. Those who practice CAM, especially licensed naturopathic medical professionals, are trained to take the time to listen. We are drilled on taking a thorough history and looking at the body as a whole system.

Most patients require a team approach because of the complexity of tick-borne infection. Typically, one medical practitioner can't be all things to a patient. Depending on the complexity of the case, both a primary care provider and a Lyme-literate doctor are often involved in patient care. Typically, there are distinct roles for each. The Lyme-literate doctor will

What We Resist, Persists: Restrictive Guidelines Limit Access to Treatment

A CONVERSATION ABOUT RESTRICTIVE GUIDELINES has to start with a brief discussion of the medical treatment guidelines commonly used to create continuity of care in the different medical specialties. These guidelines are a summary of published research, with protocols of care for many conditions seen in clinical practice across multiple specialties. Usually, medical specialists with a high level of experience and authority are chosen to be part of panels that approve them.

Guidelines can be enormously helpful—they provide a reliable process for treatment across the country, pooling information from research and clinical observed data so practitioners can best serve patients. They can also be very restrictive. The criteria currently in use to define Lyme disease are strangling open discussion, compromising funding and research, and creating scandal by maligning doctors for treating chronic Lyme disease.

IDSA Standards

The standards of care from the Infectious Diseases Society of America (IDSA) for Lyme disease, *Babesia*, and anaplasmosis are a source of contention because many practitioners, myself included, do not find the guidelines relevant to what we experience in daily practice. According to a set of guidelines titled *The Clinical Assessment, Treatment, and Prevention of Lyme Disease, Human Granulocytic Anaplasmosis, and Babesiosis: Clinical Practice Guidelines by the Infectious Diseases Society of America*[3] last updated in 2006 (these guidelines are being updated, but this process has been in the works for several years already, with no issue date yet announced):

- Appropriate measures should be taken for prevention with topical sprays, treated clothing, and tick checks.
- Medication and testing for a known tick bite is not recommended.
  - If the practitioner decided to treat, they are encouraged to give a single dose of doxycycline 200 mg.
- With the bull's-eye rash or joint pain present, it's recommended to give ten to fourteen days of antibiotic therapy, with an additional four weeks if joint swelling continues after initial treatment time.
- With neurological Lyme disease or cardiovascular infection, it's recommended to have intravenous antibiotics for fourteen to twenty-one days.
- Medications are not proven to be useful in chronic Lyme disease.
- Anaplasmosis and *Babesia* species should be suspected in those presenting with tick bite with severe illness. Treatments are recommended for ten to

fourten days. Patients are to continue to be monitored with follow-ups up to four to six months after initial treatment.

- For treatment of any Lyme disease manifestations, the following are not recommended: *"first-generation cephalosporins, fluoroquinolones, carbapenems, vancomycin, metronidazole, tinidazole, amantadine, ketolides, isoniazid, sulfamethoxazole-trimethoprim, fluconazole, benzathine penicillin G, combinations of antimicrobials, pulsed-dosing (i.e., dosing on some days but not others), long-term antibiotic therapy, anti-*Bartonella *therapies, hyperbaric oxygen, ozone, fever therapy, intravenous immunoglobulin, cholestyramine, intravenous hydrogen peroxide, specific nutritional supplements, and others"*

The last bullet point is telling. This guideline is what insurance companies use to inform their coverage. It is why, when you approach physicians about Lyme disease, many do not want to discuss alternative treatments or differing points of view. Guidelines for most conditions advise doctors what to do rather than list medications and therapies not recommended. This feature is unique to this document and explains why it has been so difficult for patients to get the help they need and to get insurance coverage for therapies. Most treatments listed here as off-limits are conventional.

The other important piece is the words at the end of the paragraph: "and others." This leaves the criteria for what is accepted and what is not very open and difficult to define. The other language is concrete, with strict limitations on treatment time and medications recommended. This does not leave a lot of room for the doctor to address the individual case with progressive options.

If you continue with symptoms beyond the current IDSA treatment recommendations, your condition is considered *Post-Lyme syndrome*. This means you are no longer treatable, according to the guidelines—you're stuck with it, and palliative medications can help manage symptoms if a prescriber agrees. Typically, language in the criteria leaves room for the doctor to exercise clinical judgment for what is best for the individual. The Centers for Disease Control (CDC) currently support and follow the standards of care laid out by the IDSA.

ILADS Standards

For every yin, there is a yang. The International Lyme and Associated Diseases Society (ILADS) was formed in 1999 by a group of practitioners from a diverse pool of specialties to create an alternative view of treatment for tick-borne infections. It's important for me to declare my bias as a member of ILADS, of which I have been a member for several years. ILADS supports preventive measures to avoid tick bites, just as the IDSA does. However, there are several differences in the guidelines of the two organizations. ILADS guidelines, titled *Evidence Assessments and Guideline Recommendations in Lyme Disease: The Clinical Management of Known Tick Bites, Erythema Migrans Rashes and Persistent Disease*[4] and published 2014, state the following:

- Clinicians should not adopt single-dose therapy with doxycycline due to low efficacy in the literature and clinical outcomes.

continued

- Treatment time for a new bite with an *Ixodes* species tick, no matter the bite time, should be treated with doxycycline 100–200 mg twice daily for twenty days.
- Education about tick bites, care with antibiotic treatment to avoid secondary infections, and prevention should be discussed in the office visit.
- "Watchful waiting" with delay in treatment *increases* risk of infection.
- Risk-to-benefit analysis shows that antibiotics need to be considered on a case-by-case basis as an opportunity for patients to regain quality of life. Withholding antibiotic therapy is costlier to the individual, the medical system, and the economy.
- Re-treatment of chronic infection should not just rely on labs but on patient reports of continued impairment related to initial infection.
- Medications and therapies should continue to evolve; practitioners should be open to what is clinically observed to be effective and safe while honoring patient choice.

Despite the efforts of both camps to stress preventive measures, the problem of tick-borne infections is continuing to grow. We need all hands on deck for this crisis. I align myself with ILADS because its criteria leave room for growth and development. This approach is needed now more than ever to find the most effective and efficient way to treat this growing problem.

handle all medications and care concerning treatment for Lyme disease, while the primary care practitioner manages health concerns unrelated to Lyme disease. The offices may run slightly differently, with varying hours of availability, definitions of practice determined by third-party insurance, and treatments that may be available.

Patients with chronic infections may require a lot of care and rehabilitation. They will typically have a physical medicine specialist, either a chiropractor or a massage therapist. Patients may benefit from attending yoga or meditation classes, and, depending on the level of physical impairment, may also be referred for formal occupational therapy or physical therapy. Many patients also have an acupuncturist to provide pain management.

If a patient experiences stress, anxiety, or depression, regular visits with a counselor can be beneficial. Experiencing chronic Lyme disease is a form of a trauma, so it's important to have proper support set up to cope. Some patients also seek out energy medicine practitioners, such as Reiki therapists, medical empaths, shamanic healers, sound healers, and biomagnetic pair therapists—just to name a few. Energy medicine offers another way to enhance the healing process, reduce pain, practice self-care, and improve well-being.

Dr. Google

ON BEHALF OF ALL DOCTORS, I would like to discuss Dr. Google. In the Lyme disease community, your search engine may be all you have if access to medical care is limited. Those with chronic health conditions are more apt to research online to learn how to manage their health, whereas the doctor used to be the primary source of information. This is a big change in a long-standing dynamic.

Far too often, however, Dr. Google's advice is chosen over that of a live doctor who knows your individual case. Once you have found a doctor, it's time to trust the process and set aside the copious research. The core issue is going to be *trusting* your health care practitioner; if you don't, find another one. Internet research can become an obsessive habit. Are you feeling empowered from the research? Are you missing out on spending time with your family or getting adequate sleep at night because of your excessive research? Do you have a medicine cabinet full of supplements you bought online because a site you found said they were going to cure Lyme disease?

Internet research is a part of the consumer-driven health care movement, but the Internet is saturated with information that has not been vetted according to any professional standards. Yet because a claim appears on the Internet, people may give it a high sense of validity. There have been many times when I felt a particular medication would be best for a patient and the patient will agree, but then he or she goes home, does some Internet research, and calls saying they found information about the medication that scares them. I will always respect a patient's choice, but it is important to ask whether the choice is being made out of fear or out of common sense. For your sanity—and for the sanity of your medical providers—it's sometimes healthy to step away from the computer.

Advocating for Yourself with Doctors

Dealing with criticism from doctors without getting derailed is difficult, but it's a valuable skill to learn. Please don't spend too much time defending yourself with a disrespectful practitioner. It's okay if a doctor does not believe chronic Lyme disease exists; just move on and find someone who is more open minded. I see many patients who want to change a doctor's mind, change the system, and convince disbelievers in the medical community that they are wrong—or they become upset by doctors who did not provide support. Focus on your healing, and then your service to making change will be in helping

Focus on your healing, and then your service to making change will be in helping others learn to advocate for themselves.

others learn to advocate for themselves. I know many of you have been through humiliating discussions, had invasive procedures, and been prescribed medications that did not help. Holding on to anger just feeds the illness. It's okay to be angry at the disjointed system, but try to let your anger move through you to resolution instead of holding on to it.

What is truly important? That you work with practitioners who have an open mind, a compassionate heart, and patience with your process. Find a proper support system of practitioners from different modalities: a Lyme-literate doctor, a primary care practitioner linked with the hospital system, a specialist (if needed) for other diagnoses being medically managed, a chiropractor, a massage therapist, a counselor, support groups, an energy medicine practitioner, and a naturopathic doctor. Not all may have experience with Lyme disease, but they can still provide valuable care to help you heal.

When you are approaching your primary care provider about Lyme disease, be aware that in almost every state doctors are mandated by hospital regulations to run the two-tiered testing for Lyme disease; they may not be able to run a Western blot. In addition to requesting tests to confirm Lyme disease, ask to have coinfection tests run. Depending on the state where you live, you may not have insurance coverage for a naturopathic doctor or a Lyme-literate specialist if the doctor is out of network. You can ask your primary care provider to work with your Lyme specialist to run labs for coverage as needed. A handful of patients in my practice have HMOs that require them to get a referral from their primary care provider to see a specialist.

It's important to keep all doctors you are working with fully informed by sharing lab work and reporting all medications you are taking, including supplements. It is critical, for your safety, to avoid medication interactions. In addition to medicines that may interact in a dangerous way, many supplements can have adverse reactions with pharmaceutical medications. You may be nervous to tell a medical doctor you are treating Lyme disease or using alternative medications. Many doctors may not understand the training of a naturopathic doctor and have varying opinions about the naturopathic doctor's ability to practice medicine. They may also not agree with the treatment of Lyme disease, especially if you are working with a rheumatologist or neurologist who believes your issues are due to a different diagnosis. Talking with your medical doctors about Lyme disease may be uncomfortable, but it is important. I encourage transparency in my treatment plan and leave an open door of communication with all other practitioners who work with my patient.

As a general rule, when working with more than one practitioner, only one doctor should be prescribing medications for the tick-borne infections. You can have a different specialist who may prescribe pain management medications, blood sugar–regulating medications, or medications to manage elevated blood pressure. To maintain the integrity of your treatment, leave the prescribing of antibiotics and those medications related specifically to Lyme disease to one person. This is my rule if a patient is seeing other practitioners who parallel my specialty, such as a Lyme-literate M.D. I am perfectly fine managing the natural medication protocols but will not be involved in prescribing antibiotics.

Finally, do not be afraid to be assertive. As I said before, it is okay if your doctor does not believe you. It is fine if your doctor does not agree with your treatment choice, as long as the provider is professional and compassionate. Speak up for what you want in terms of your health care. Remember, the doctors work for you. Doctors have to set proper boundaries to maintain professional expectations and ensure safety within their scope of practice, but your opinion on your health care matters. Your treatment needs to match your values and beliefs and must meet you where you are in life to be truly successful.

Chronic Tick-Borne Disease Is a Family Affair

Social support is one of the most important parts of recovery for Lyme patients, who frequently feel abandoned by their family and community. Being supported is not just about having physical help; it is about being able to go through the recovery process without having to explain or defend the illness. Lyme patients need to be able to have the recovery process take the time it takes and feel unconditionally loved, especially by their family.

The fact that recovery times are more than a year makes Lyme disease very difficult on caretakers as well as on sufferers. Services or support systems must be in place for all involved. When someone is first diagnosed, I assess for social support, physical support, and the general sentiment in the household. Is there good communication between parties? Does the caretaker or loved one believe the patient has Lyme disease? Does the family communicate with compassion? Is an overabundance of worry placed on the patient? How much fear is there? Is the person expected to get well too quickly? Is the patient coddled to the point that it is hindering progress? Is the patient treating his family well or showing poor emotional control?

Often, a Lyme disease patient feels she is a burden to loved ones, and this feeling can lead to deep depression. Depression reduces immunity, decreases quality of life, and fuels suicidal ideation in many. The truth is, Lyme disease is a family affair. If a person is debilitated with Lyme disease, the entire family dynamic will change—physically, mentally, emotionally, and financially. This change affects the marriage, parent-child relationships, financial plans, job standings, and the quality of family life.

An interesting phenomenon is that, though chronic Lyme disease is well known in the media, in communities with epidemics, and within families, people still tend to be wary of discussing their illness with others. They do not tend to share the fact that they are struggling with Lyme disease with others in their life. When I say "they," I mean not only the patient but also the whole family. The stress of Lyme disease is extremely difficult to handle for spouses, children, and extended family, as well as the patient. Damage is done when a person feels the need to hide physical, mental, and emotional pain because he doesn't want to be a bother, and when he resists being honest about suffering to spare others stress. Lyme disease patients may fear being judged by others and worry that friends or relatives think they are making up symptoms or milking the situation.

Start by being authentic about how you feel and letting go of the shame associated with having Lyme disease. Recovery is a difficult process, and you will need to process emotions so stress does not build up. It's especially important to make space for emotional release and to have healthy outlets such as meditation, yoga, prayer time, writing time, and even crying time. Crying loosens what is tied too tight. Let the tears flow if they arise. Then share your feelings with others if you need to. Realize they can't fix all your ills, but they can listen and hold space for you to process. This is also about cultivating healthy boundaries for all involved so that expectations are clear about how much a person can give and also what you would like to receive.

Seeing a counselor who can work both with you individually and with the family can be a healthy way to address the stress from the get-go by developing healthy communication and coping mechanisms. You'll need to have an understanding in the household about the importance of creating an environment suitable for healing with adequate rest, nutrition, and stability throughout the process.

It's also essential for the mental stability of the Lyme disease patient that she is believed. A person can more easily face disbelief in the medical community or at work if loved ones reflect unconditional support. If this is not the case, recovery can be much more traumatizing and prolonged. Believing the impact of the Herxheimer reaction (discussed in chapter 6) is also vital—for patients of all ages. It's incredibly painful for the symptoms to be dismissed as an authentic response to the infection.

Support groups are popping up all over, driven by a grassroots movement to help those who are struggling. Meetings are typically held at churches, libraries, health clinics, and individuals' homes. They can offer a welcoming place where you do not need to explain what you are going through; it's already understood. Meeting others who feel as you do is helpful in dealing with the loneliness and isolation of the disease, and in assuring you that your process is normal. Cultivating supportive relationships is also wonderful for the immune system!

Representing Yourself to Workplaces and Schools

Working while recovering from Lyme disease and coinfections is very difficult. You may feel pressure to stay employed, be seen as competent, and avoid discrimination, depending on the sentiment toward the disease in your workplace. Many people do not have flexibility to take time off from work or a guarantee that their job will be waiting for them. If you hide the fact you're sick yet your performance suffers, you could lose your job based on the perception you are not capable or committed.

To protect yourself at work, document your illness if it is chronic and requires long-term treatment. This is usually done through paperwork associated with the Family and Medical Leave Act. Though there are a number of caveats and eligibility requirements, this federal law can protect the individual who is ill and a caretaker who will require time off work. You will be able to report your diagnosis, prognosis, and treatment, and make accommodations for more frequent breaks as needed and approved time off for doctor's appointments. This is another way to help support your recovery and be transparent with your employer while protecting your job.

Pressure similar to that placed on adult employees can affect children, who tend to want to keep the illness secret and try to keep up the pace at school, without much success. Teachers who don't know the child is ill may think parents are just not following through by monitoring homework and study time. Poor performance on tests or assignments can lead to the child being penalized, which just creates a more difficult environment in which to succeed. Kids can lose confidence, which is difficult to recover from at a young age.

Paperwork commonly done to help with accommodations for school include 504 plans and individualized education plans (IEPs). These plans are made in conjunction with parents, school personnel, and the medical practitioner and can help by making absences excused, evaluating ways the school staff can help the student be more successful, providing more time to complete work, and designating alternative testing environments to aid concentration. Nursing staff within schools have been helpful in administering doses of probiotics or supplements for my patients as needed.

Lyme Denial: Delaying the Inevitable

An all too common phenomenon among Lyme disease patients is denial of the disease. Some patients call the clinic, panicked that they have Lyme disease and anxious to get an appointment as soon as possible. A few weeks later the flare subsides, and they cancel the appointment because they are all better. A month later, they are sick again with a flare and call in a panic, upset they missed the original appointment and wanting another one. This pattern sometimes repeats several times before I meet a patient, maybe a year later.

Many people will meet with me to be tested, or to have their children tested, for tick-borne infection. After I take the history of the patient and decide that there is enough evidence to support the idea of testing, I order the necessary tests. If the results are positive, I report them, but often the patient calls the office to say he believes he doesn't have the infection. This is absolutely his prerogative, and it's his right not to pursue treatment. Yet, several months later we will get a call from the patient, who comes in reporting how sick he has been, and how afraid he was once he spoke with his primary care doctor and showed the doctor the results. After seeing his health decline over time, the patient is finally ready to move forward with treatment. Most patients who enter this cycle experience regret about waiting so long and fear they will not recover.

Sick children with parents who do not get along, such as those who are separated or divorced, can also face difficulty when it's time to decide on treatment. Many children have one parent who spends more time with the child and who feels the child requires treatment. The other parent (whom I typically don't meet) believes the child is fine because there is no such thing as chronic Lyme disease. The child stays sick because both parents must agree on the plan in order to move forward productively. Even if treatment begins, maintaining regular doses of medications can be difficult, depending on who the child is staying with at the time. It's a complicated situation for all involved.

Doctor-hopping is another common behavior, rooted in the desire to find a magic pill that will cure all. Patients become frustrated as they search for a treatment that will bring an end to suffering in the same time frame that they would recover from a routine infection. This leads them to jump on and off protocols, move from one doctor to the next, self-treat, and try many different options, often abandoning them before they would reasonably have a chance to work. I feel this tendency has to do with the fear of experiencing discomfort with treatment—patients feeling unsettled and worry they are making the wrong choice—and they think the next treatment will be the answer they are looking for. They may become concerned they are missing out on the "cure" if they stay too long with a treatment that doesn't work immediately, or they worry that discomfort the current treatment causes means it's not right for them. Hopping from doctor to doctor and abandoning treatments can also be motivated by a partner, family members, or the parent of a patient. People want to be well—and they want their loved ones to be well—and many try multiple avenues, exhausting themselves chasing a cure.

You *can* heal from tick-borne disease. This may mean letting go of the person you used to be and accepting changes that may be permanent, but in most cases, you can dramatically increase your quality of life.

On the flip side, it's important to have a team approach to blending treatment modalities. Changing your treatment strategy may be the right choice for you, and it's essential that you have providers from different specialties available to help, but jumping from one to another does not help you get well. Recovery from chronic tick-borne disease takes time, patience, and persistence. Doctor-hopping behavior is much different from moving on from a treatment if it's not the right fit. Just be aware of your goal as you decide to stop a protocol. Are you making the choice out of fear or placing all your hopes on a promised cure that seems too good to be true?

You *can* heal from tick-borne disease. This may mean letting go of the person you used to be and accepting changes that may be permanent, but in most cases, you can dramatically increase your quality of life. I do not promise a cure because that would be misleading. A specific protocol may be one person's answer but not work on the next, and finding the right treatment is sometimes a matter of trial and error.

Finding the right treatment takes time, patience, and trust in the journey. It's not easy. As a medical professional, I get frustrated at times if an infection does not resolve in the way I was hoping. There are many ups and downs sitting in the doctor's chair, as I see one patient feeling on top of the world and the next in misery.

When I was a patient years ago, I had many emotional meltdowns and questioned everything I was doing, including my career choice. If I could not recover using the approach I recommended to patients, then what was I doing with my life? I experienced all the same emotions I saw in my patients. It took me two years of treatment, blending medications, physical medicine, and energy medicine. I learned a lot from being a patient, and that experience has been very helpful in my ability to treat others—this was one of the gifts the healing process provided me.

In Summary

You are not alone—and my goal is to make sure you know this. Remember, the politics around Lyme disease denial is not a personal attack—it's bigger than your individual case. This perspective allows you to release the burden of defending yourself. Be prepared to face scrutiny for a while longer, until this disease is better understood and given the compassion it deserves. Know that others around you are experiencing the same challenges. Once you have recovered, you can be the voice in another sufferer's ear to nudge them to investigate Lyme disease and provide them with compassion as you share your journey. You can help another person with Lyme disease advocate for himself and bring your greater perspective to reduce his suffering.

CHAPTER 6

SETTING THE STAGE FOR TREATMENT SUCCESS

T aking the leap into treatment is difficult given the amount of fear surrounding a diagnosis of Lyme disease, the complicated politics, and the need to weed through mounds of information with discernment. In this chapter, I'll address choosing the right supplements to make your treatment plan sustainable. We'll also look at the overall costs of Lyme disease, what to expect with treatment, and how to structure your day with a medication regimen—and we'll take a deeper look at the Herxheimer reaction.

Choosing the Right Supplements

Not all products marketed to treat Lyme disease are as promised. Some make big claims without delivering, while others are overpriced given the ingredients they contain. Navigating treatment protocols can be difficult as you try to choose one that is affordable and that you think you will be able to follow consistently, while avoiding becoming overwhelmed by the options. You want the best out of your

As a consumer, it's important to ask what research backs up the claims being made about a treatment or a product.

medications but may not want to take so many supplements that you are consuming more pills than you are food in a day. At that point, you are digesting more fillers and binders than nutrients from those supplements. Most patients eventually reject treatment altogether because of pill fatigue.

If your supplement list fills an entire page, you may need to pare it down. Patients come to my clinic with a grocery bag full of supplements they've bought based on Internet research. This is known as *polypharmacy* (concurrent use of multiple medications) with supplements. It's easy to become excited by promises found online and feel hopeful that this supplement will be the magic pill that will get you to the finish line quickly. The reality of tick-borne disease is that treatment will involve taking more pills than you ever thought possible for longer than you ever imagined, but moderation is still vital.

It's important, too, to be conscious of the exact herb you are purchasing and to be aware whom you are buying it from and whether the plant cultivation is sustainable. Many people are turning to large resale vendors to buy supplements rather than purchasing them directly from the company or a doctor. This tendency is motivated mainly by the urge to be frugal, which is understandable; but it is important to ask how the independent seller has been storing the supplement and for how long. The product may be cheaper, but it may be a bargain because a seller wants to unload it. If the supplement is expired or has not been stored properly, it may not carry the same potency.

Lyme disease patients and their families obviously want to get well as soon as possible, which makes them vulnerable to marketing promises and anecdotal information. The FDA does not allow supplement companies to make structure-function claims—this means that a company cannot say on the bottle or in its marketing material that a particular supplement treats a disease. It cannot say the supplement "treats ulcers" or "treats rheumatoid arthritis";[1] instead, it may say something to the effect that the supplement "supports healthy digestion" or "reduces inflammation." As a consumer, it's important to ask what research backs up the claims being made about a treatment or a product. Who paid for the research, and have other studies replicated the results? Nothing and no one should be boasting they will cure you. This is not to say statements such as this will not be made, but please question the ethics and motives of someone who comes forth with such claims.

Patients in the Lyme disease community are exceptionally vulnerable because they are desperate to recover. Many herbs and nutraceuticals have proven themselves over time with observed data and beneficial outcomes. Treatment needs to align with your life: to what you can commit to doing on a daily basis, what you can afford, and what aligns with your values. It's important to consider the risks and the benefits of any treatment path you choose.

Chronic Lyme Disease Has No Quick Fix

We live in a culture that has limited patience for a body facing illness and recovery. It has been about six years since my bout of chronic Lyme disease and babesiosis, but while I was writing this book, I had a dream. I was walking around my house feeling panicked that my symptoms were back. In the dream, I had a thought that calmed me down: "Maybe now that Lyme disease is back, I can get more rest."

I woke up to realize I was not having a relapse, but I was left with the dream's message: I was overextended. I was not making enough time for myself. My unconscious mind knew it would get my attention with the idea I could be having a relapse. I bring this up because many patients resist rest and are angry with the body for not getting well soon enough. They will literally be brought to their knees before they make changes in their schedule that allow them to recuperate. As they try to maintain the same work or school load and social activities, they get even more aggravated with the body and resist the need to simplify their lives. This resistance to making changes prolongs the healing process, and the body is aware of the anger, responding with reduced energy and lower healing capacity.

The average treatment time for chronic Lyme disease is six months to a year. Treatment for an acute bite lasts only three to four weeks. These dramatically different treatment times illustrate why it is so important to treat a bite as soon as possible. It takes longer than you would think to recover from chronic Lyme disease, and this fact will trip you up more than any other. I talk daily with people who wonder whether they really do have Lyme disease, since they are not well in two months.

Doubts surface as inner conflict, as you ask the following questions: "Am I sure this is really Lyme disease?" "Is it okay that my recovery is taking so long?" "Should I change treatment, see a new specialist, stop treatment?" Then someone in your daily life asks you these questions in passing, reinforcing your insecurity and creating more frustration. Maybe a new treatment will get you to the finish line faster? You might get stuck mentally between a fear of moving forward and a fear of stopping. You will hit the wall many times, with discomfort and impatience with the process. This is all normal. Understanding that your thought process is typical and that you are not alone will hopefully help calm your mental chatter.

Family members and friends, with all the best intentions, may also step in to give advice. They might know a person who was cured by this supplement, or they might offer the opinion that you don't have Lyme disease, based on their own Internet research. They might feel the same frustration you do as they watch someone they care for suffering.

Once you start treatment, the first two to four months are the most difficult. Symptom flares might be at their worst then, with the remainder of treatment time featuring random flares as treatment gets to different layers in the body. It takes time for toxins to be released and inflammation to subside. You can expect to see improvement of most symptoms over time but will continue to have difficult moments and require time for your health to be fully restored. You will know you are close to finishing treatment when you forget for a while that you are sick or when two months go by with no symptom flare. You may also see symptom flares gradually become less severe and shorter in duration.

A phenomenon I refer to as the "four-month slump" commonly occurs partway through treatment; during this slump, it feels as if you've taken twenty steps backward in the treatment process. This usually hits patients hardest if they were one of the lucky ones who saw immediate improvement with antibiotics. I feel this happens because of a release of spirochetes that were dormant in the cyst form, causing a dramatic Herxheimer reaction. As we discussed earlier, Lyme disease spirochetes live in four different forms, one of which, the cyst form, is shaped like a ball. This reaction does not occur with everyone, but it is fairly normal. A slump or plateau may also indicate that you are due for a dosage change, which is something to broach with your treating physician.

You may have a relapse or a flare well after treatment is complete. This usually happens when either you were infected by new tick bite or you experience a major stressor that jars the immune system. Stressors can be another illness, a car accident, a devastating loss, a concussion, a sports injury, or surgery; these events can place enough shock on the body that Lyme disease resurfaces. Coinfections missed with the first round of treatment can also be the culprit. Most cases are likely new bites.

Lyme disease recovery is a time to slow down and listen to what your body needs. You must learn how to say no and work on any feelings of guilt that arise when you step away from your typical pace. Lyme disease has its own timetable. Once you accept and understand this, you will experience great relief. Note that doctors get just as tripped up by this anxious energy because we want to see patients recover as quickly as possible. I have had to learn to manage the emotions of coping with patients' ups and downs without taking their progress personally. A consistent meditative practice and energy hygiene practice make this much easier. The less attached I am to the patient recovering within a certain time frame, the healthier the process is for the patient. I don't need to be another person adding to the patient's stress over expectations; instead, I work to truly hold space for the patient to be authentic with the experience.

The Cost of Lyme Disease

Lyme disease is not your average infection, with loads of money being poured into research; in fact, the opposite is happening. Considering the impact tick-borne disease is having on communities across the globe, federal and state governing bodies are spending very little to educate citizens, track the disease process in humans, or research prevention and treatments for the disease. Currently, the funding provided by federal and local governments in states most affected is barely enough to pay for staff to track reported cases in local Health and Human Services offices.

Around 2013, the Centers for Disease Control updated its reporting, giving the number of infected persons in the United States per year as 300,000 rather than the long-reported number of approximately 30,000 people. To put this in perspective, there are 1.5 percent more Lyme disease cases each year than there are breast cancer cases (200,000) and the rate of infection with Lyme is six times higher than infection with HIV (50,000), as reported in 2014. Chronic Lyme disease patients visit doctors five times more often and emergency rooms twice as often as the average population.[2]

Socioeconomically, it's costing us all a lot to deny the presence of chronic Lyme disease in the population. We are seeing increased numbers of disability claims, higher health care costs, lower quality of life, reduced productivity at work, and missed days of school. And we are looking at an enormous increase in chronic disease in the population, which will be an ongoing economic problem. It's estimated that 42 percent of chronic Lyme disease patients cannot work during their treatment, which means lost wages for the patient as well as out-of-pocket expenses due to high deductibles and rejected claims, plus costs for supportive treatments such as supplements. This can cost, on average, $1,000 to $2,000 per month out of pocket for patients who have medical insurance.

I spend a fair amount of time each week filling out disability forms and Family and Medical Leave Act paperwork, on the phone advocating for patients with insurance companies, and submitting prior authorizations for insurance coverage for medications. Many people are forced to leave their jobs either to be a caretaker to a family member with chronic Lyme disease or to care for themselves as they are suffering from Lyme disease and are not well enough to manage at work. Most of these patients had been working full time in well-paying professions with healthy retirement funds that they must drain to pay for treatment such as intravenous medications that are typically not covered by insurance companies.

In addition, there is the cost of palliative medications, lab tests, doctor's visits, and therapies for symptom management. Many patients require medications to support the cardiovascular system, manage pain, balance blood sugar, lower cholesterol, and control attention deficit disorder, as well as anti-inflammatories and mood stabilizers—and the list goes on. My patients usually have a list of five or more pharmaceuticals to report on the first visit, based on all the doctors they have seen before coming to me. They spend large amounts of money on blood tests, imaging studies, surgeries, medications, and experimental treatments for other diagnoses before they are tested for Lyme disease; Lyme disease is usually last on the list.

I never could understand the logic of denying antibiotics to someone who is living in an area infested with disease-bearing ticks and who has several questionable symptoms. It is especially bewildering if the onset of symptoms was sudden. It is much more affordable to treat with a short course of antibiotics and then, if necessary, escalate to more extensive testing to confirm other conditions that involve long-term care. The cost of an antibiotic is low when compared with the cost of palliative care for chronic conditions.

The most high-cost issue with tick-borne disease patients is the number of hospital and clinic visits they require. Most patients report frequent emergency room visits for chest pain and heart palpitations. Others go because of vertigo, elevated body pain, and severe depression or anxiety. Most will be given a sedative in the emergency room and sent home with a diagnosis of anxiety. Many are treated like drug seekers or leave feeling dumbfounded that doctors found nothing wrong, though they feel so sick. On more than one occasion, patients say an emergency room doctor handed my name and number to them, suggesting they contact me for help.

Maintaining the Medication Schedule

If you are not used to taking medications, I'm sorry to tell you that you may need to take more than you are comfortable with if you are to recover fully. Eventually, however, the plan is to be off them altogether. Chronic Lyme disease patients are often taking a long list of prescription medications before their first appointment with me. Most common are those for mood stability, inflammation, and pain management, as well as antiallergy medications, antacids, antibiotics, immunosuppressants for autoimmune symptoms, blood pressure stabilizers, antiseizure medications, cholesterol-lowering medications, sleep aids, and blood sugar regulators. Often, more than one prescriber is involved.

One of the biggest difficulties in maintaining compliance with treatment is finding a dosing schedule that does not feel burdensome. This is most difficult for individuals who hate taking pills but who now must take them several times in a day. For treatment to be successful, you will need to make sure you lay out a plan for your daily life that allows your medication regimen to be sustainable. I learned the hard way, through my own two years of treatment, how easy it is to forget a dose. My children were very young when I had Lyme disease, and I was easily distracted by their needs. I would come back a couple of hours later to find my medications still on the counter. I found it was easiest to plan dosing around mealtimes; this timing is conducive to a daily flow and feels less intrusive.

When I'm working to devise a patient's treatment plan, I first check in with the needs of the family. For instance, if the patient is a child, I need to find a dosing schedule that works for the parents and within the school schedule. If multiple children in the family are being treated at the same time (which happens far too often), the parents and I need to coordinate care in order to avoid burnout. I also need to make sure the process is structured so that dosing is consistent.

The same considerations apply for adults. In many situations, a patient may not have the cognitive ability to remember to take medications regularly and must depend on reminders such as cell phone alarms, family support, or lists; most end up using pillboxes with the medications laid out daily. Lyme disease patients also tend to have irregular sleep cycles, which makes regular meals and consistent dosing difficult. Following are typical recommendations for dosing:

- Take your antibiotics at breakfast and dinnertime. Some antibiotics may need to be taken at least thirty minutes before eating. Remember that certain antibiotics, such as doxycycline (the most popular Lyme disease medication) and minocycline, should not be taken with food, dairy products, or mineral supplements because of the reduced absorption of the medication. In this case, it's best to take your medication thirty minutes to an hour before your meal. Please check the prescription bottle for special instructions from the

Herxheimer Reaction

JARISCH-HERXHEIMER REACTION, often referred to as simply a Herxheimer reaction or Herxing, is a common phenomenon in the treatment of tick-borne infections. It's named after two scientists who recognized a unique reaction in their patients while treating syphilis, another spirochete infection, in the early 1900s. As the spirochetes are attacked by medications or the host's immune system, endotoxins are released, increasing inflammation in the area where the pathogen is located. This can occur in multiple organ systems, making it difficult for patients to tolerate the medication due to increased body pain, neurological symptoms, headaches, fatigue, fevers, mood instability, and rashes. Unfortunately, this reaction is the rule rather than the exception. It can happen within a few hours of initiating treatment or may be as delayed as four weeks. The reaction can last several months, with the worst typically happening within the first two to four months of starting treatment. A Herxheimer reaction is the number one reason people stop treatment, and the fear of this reaction can stop people cold at the thought of being unable to work or take care of their family. Supporting patients emotionally as well as physically through the process is the most important factor in treatment success.

The intensity of the Herxheimer reaction depends on how long the infection has been with the patient, how many other tick-borne infections are present in the body, how well the patient's detox pathways are working, and how much the patient fears suffering. Patients who have a history of unresolved mental, emotional, or physical abuse can have greater difficulty because they may feel victimized all over again when the pain increases. The reaction can trigger post-traumatic stress disorder, leading to intense fear and anxiety. Patients may experience a fight-or-flight response at just the thought of taking treatment, including flashbacks, panic attacks, and emotions so intense they can have thoughts of self-harm. Patients may benefit from a referral to a counselor who specializes in trauma. For most people to recover, they must tolerate treatment consistently over time.

Symptoms will come and go periodically, sometimes varying with the hour or the day. The infection is turning the corner when the flares are less severe and less frequent; eventually, there are days when the patient forgets she is sick. Disappearance of symptoms becomes the benchmark for identifying the end of therapy. Over the years, my criterion for stopping treatment has been two months with no symptoms related to Lyme disease or other coinfections. It's also important to understand that the Herxheimer reaction can occur in response to other situations as well: when the body is clearing toxins such as yeast overgrowth, when fasting, or during chelation therapy for heavy metals intoxication. This means the treatment plan must always support detoxification pathways by including toxin-binding supplements and nutrients that encourage the production of glutathione, a potent detoxifier made by the liver.

Below are tips to support you through the process:

- Remain calm. Every symptom you have had that is related to your tick-borne illness could amplify. Symptoms may come and go in irregular patterns. Rest as much as you can.
- Stay well hydrated and set a goal of drinking half your body weight in ounces of filtered water each day.
- Take a sauna (set the temperature to 120°F [49°C] and start for five minutes; gradually work your way up to fifteen to twenty minutes).
- Soak in a bath to which you've added two cups of Epsom; this will help the body in removing toxins.
- Take Alka-Seltzer Gold (for those over nineteen years of age because it contains aspirin) or electrolyte powders added to water. This remedy can reduce headaches and nausea, improve clarity and energy, and relieve mild body pain. Use as directed and as needed for support.
- Take liposomal glutathione, one teaspoon one or two times daily by mouth or of 1–2 g two or three times per week administered intravenously. Glutathione is a powerful antioxidant that is important to the body's detox process; it supplements a protein compound already made by the body in the combination of L-glycine, L-cysteine, and glycine.
- Practice meditation or do gentle yoga to promote a balanced nervous system and healthy blood flow, which will help remove toxins.
- Recognize that it is normal to experience a Herxheimer reaction with Lyme disease and other tick-borne infections. While the reaction may not be perceived as normal by others, know that it is common.

pharmacy. If you still have questions, contact your doctor or pharmacist to confirm proper timing. A majority of antibiotics are preferably taken with food to avoid nausea and help in absorption.

- Take your supplements at lunchtime and before bed. This schedule keeps a healthy distance between doses of your probiotics and antibiotics, which will give you the best outcome. It also breaks up the number of pills you must take at one time, so your digestive tract is not overwhelmed.
- Work with your prescribing doctor to factor in timing of any other prescription medications you are taking. A common medication is thyroid replacement, which requires dosing first thing in the morning, one hour away from food or other medications.

What patients *don't* know...can lead to impulsive decisions and panic, causing harm in the end.

Don't worry if you miss a dose. You have not screwed anything up if your day does not work out the way you wanted and doses aren't perfectly timed. If you can, try to fit the missed dose in later, but not at the cost of lost sleep or the digestive upset that may come when you take too much medication at once. Just start over again the next day. If scheduling mishaps happen frequently, discuss your dosing timetable with your prescriber so you can rework it in a way that better suits your life.

In Summary

You are now better prepared for treatment of chronic tick-borne infection. The information in this chapter is meant to empower you, encourage you to stay the course with treatment, and learn to troubleshoot situations as they arise. I find that what patients *don't* know—the experiences they have that they fear aren't normal—can lead to impulsive decisions and panic, causing harm in the end. An open dialogue about recovery makes the process more tolerable. Next, we will discuss the Foundational Naturopathic Treatment Plan, the nuts and bolts of the most important supplements to support the physical body through the recovery process.

CHAPTER 7

THE FOUNDATIONAL NATUROPATHIC TREATMENT PLAN

T he Foundational Naturopathic Treatment Plan is about sustainability during a difficult recovery process: A treatment is not worthwhile if a patient is unable to comply either physically or financially. My requirements are that a treatment plan be reasonably priced for the majority of patients, easy to implement, and proven safe and effective. It needs to help patients feel more hopeful without making over-the-top claims of a cure.

Treating Lyme disease and associated infections is a big subject. There are so many different protocols that exploring the best options can feel truly overwhelming. Over the years, I have seen many treatment fads for Lyme disease come and go, and at this stage in my medical career I'm discerning about what I implement in my practice. My goal is to give you an understanding of options for treatment. I have honed this plan not only as a naturopathic doctor but as a Lyme disease patient who had to work medications into the flow of my life. The treatment goals I have for each patient are as follows:

- Reduce inflammation and pain.
- Treat the infections with a blend of complementary medications.

- Balance the hormone system with nutrients, herbs, and bioidentical hormones.
- Improve detoxification pathways by supporting organs of elimination and greening your life.
- Boost immunity through herbal support, stress management, and proper nutrient balance.
- Balance mood, increase clarity of thought, and promote empowerment and sleep regularity to improve well-being.
- Support a heathy digestive tract.
- Improve strength and endurance with movement.

Whichever direction you choose—either blending natural medication with antibiotics or taking natural medications only—I want to provide you with a foundation to build on and maintain a healthy physical structure to make healing more efficient. Whether the option I present stands alone as your primary therapy or in combination with other modalities, these options should be at the core of helping you restore your health. In the back of the book, you'll find a handy reference section with charts that detail the herbs and nutrients discussed in this chapter.

Maintaining a Healthy Microbiome

Trillions upon trillions of microbes colonize the tissues of our bodies, both internally and externally, and a diverse microbiome contains protective yeast, parasites, and viruses as well as bacteria. These microbes are our guards at the gates. They protect us by secreting their own antimicrobial substances to ward off invaders, educating our immune system and balancing inflammatory responses to aid in healing. These microbes change depending on the needs of the body.

The Human Microbiome Project, started in 2007 by the National Institutes of Health, was pivotal in gaining an understanding of the complexity and diversity of the microbes living in our inner world. Before this initiative, many microbes could not be isolated or cultured outside the body with an external medium. Bacteria, funguses, protozoa, bacteriophages (viruses living on bacteria), and other viruses make up a whole universe living within the human body in a co-creative relationship. The human body hosts more than ten times the number of microbial cells as it has human cells, and the Human

Microbiome Project uses genetic sequencing to understand microbes, their role in human health, and the strains that are more prevalent in certain groups. The more we understand how microbes interrelate and how they relate to the human body, the more we understand ourselves.

Maintaining healthy microflora is one of the most important aspects of treatment in every infectious disease treatment protocol. Every patient I treat is on a high-dose probiotic to combat the risks of developing yeast overgrowth or a more dangerous infection, *Clostridium difficile*. *C. difficile* is most commonly picked up in medical facilities, but it can be acquired elsewhere. Those over the age of sixty-five are most at risk for severe consequences as a result of age-related immune compromise. With proper amounts of probiotics and beneficial yeast, these infections can be avoided. I have seen only three cases of *C. difficile* in more than a decade of practice, though I have used antibiotics to treat several thousand patients with tick-borne disease. I attribute this to proper support of the human microflora.

Once relegated to health food stores, probiotics have become a household word, with big companies adding them to yogurts and other foods, and chain stores stocking them in the vitamin aisles. There are many probiotics on the market, with the main bacterial components of these being *Lactobacillus* and *Bifidobacterium*. Some cultures found in probiotics at the health food store seem as if they are infections—*Streptococcus*, for example—but they are actually part of a healthy microbiome, and the treatment goal is to promote several different strains. For many of the nonbeneficial microbes we come into contact with, there exists a beneficial microbial counterpart. We have a germ-phobic culture, but it's important to understand that approximately 98 percent of microbes are not harmful.[1] Globally, they are responsible for oxygen production, soil regeneration, degradation of toxins, and fermentation of commonly consumed foods.[2]

Each human gut has a diverse microbial population, the makeup of which depends on early life exposure to microbes, health status, genetics, and local environmental factors. Your gut is one giant "super organism," and without it, you would be unable to tolerate food without experiencing repeated infections. Although the gut is within the body, it faces outward, like the skin, with microbes living both within the body and on the surface of the skin. The microbiome is a layer coating the surface of the digestive tract, our oral cavity, the vaginal canal in women, our sinuses, under our fingernails, and on the surface of our skin, with different pathogens colonizing specific areas depending on the requirements of the body. Beneficial microbes are responsible for vitamin production, neurohormone production, mood regulation, food cravings, and immune regulation affecting gene expression; and they inform us about the outside world. When we travel, we are exposed to new microbes,

Microbes:
Friends with Benefits

PEOPLE WORLDWIDE ARE INCREASINGLY INTERESTED in delving into their genetics, so why not also get to know the micro-friends that are unique to you? Each individual has a distinctive set of microbes, a bit like each has a unique fingerprint, with more than a thousand species living in the human gut. If you want to know more about your own gut ecology, I highly recommend taking the Ubiome test (www.ubiome.com) or the Gut Zoomer by Vibrant Wellness.

Laboratories test the human microbiome either by looking at the 16S rDNA, a protein subunit present in every microbe that helps identify the microbe's origin, or through metagenomics, which tells us more about the role microbes play in the human microbiome. Depending on the test, you can get an idea of the microbes within your digestive tract or, if you're a woman, your vaginal flora. These tests can be very helpful in getting answers about persistent constipation, diarrhea, bloating, inability to lose weight, and many other troublesome problems. It's important to know more about the trillions of microbes that live with us daily and protect against invaders, produce vitamins, and regulate metabolic function. They are our friends with benefits.

which help us adjust to the new environment. Even in our own environment, the incoming microbes share information and increase our adaptability to our environment by informing the immune system.[3]

SUPPLEMENTING WITH PROBIOTICS

Ideally, a probiotic will have at least 50 billion to 150 billion colony-forming units (CFUs) per capsule to minimize the number of pills that must be taken in a day. Many of the brands on health food store shelves will have doses ranging from one million to twenty billion CFUs per capsule, which is perfect for a routine daily health regimen but not suitable to take with antibiotic therapy. The higher-CFU probiotics can be more expensive than the ones found at the grocery store, but it's worth the price to avoid side effects.

In addition to over-the-counter products, there are prescription probiotics with four hundred to nine hundred billion CFUs per dose in sachet packets. These mega-dose probiotics—including VSL #3, VSL Double Strength (DS), UltraFlora by Metagenics, and Ultimate Flora by Renew

Life—were developed for more severe intestinal inflammatory disorders such as Crohn's disease and ulcerative colitis. I often recommend doses this high, but it's important to discuss specifics with your provider; be sure probiotics are included in your treatment plan if an antibiotic is part of the course of treatment for tick-borne disease.

Note that, because most probiotics should be refrigerated, people often miss their dose in the middle of the day if they aren't at home or don't have a refrigerator at work. The probiotics I recommend are stable at room temperature for five to nine days, but brands vary in their recommendations. It's okay to bring your probiotics with you during the day in your purse or in a pill case so you can get your lunchtime dose. Consistency makes a big difference in the long run.

SUPPLEMENTING WITH PREBIOTICS

Inulin, glucomannan, and fructo-oligosaccharides (FOS) are known as *prebiotics*, and are frequently given alongside a probiotics regimen. Prebiotics help feed the beneficial bacteria in the digestive tract, supporting them as they do their job of supporting you. Research has shown that konjac glucomannan, a prebiotic fiber supplement, provides protective benefit to the important gut microbe *Bifidobacterium*, the most abundant beneficial microbes in the human body.

Glucomannan protects native *Bifidobacterium* when patients are being treated with the antibiotics tetracycline, streptomycin, and penicillin.[4] This is due to the ability of konjac glucomannan to absorb toxins that would harm *Bifidobacterium*. This prebiotic would be helpful as an addition to your probiotic regimen while on treatment; the usual dose is one-quarter to one-half teaspoon added to water one or two times per day. Inulin and FOS have also been shown to decrease the symptoms associated with irritable bowel syndrome, Crohn's disease, and ulcerative colitis.[5] A common side effect of prebiotics is bloating, which typically resolves over time as the gut adapts.

EATING A FLORA-SUPPORTIVE DIET

Since the beginning of time, the environment has provided biodiverse microbial species that colonize the human body. Our first exposure is from our mothers in the birth canal; then we are exposed through breast milk, family pets, other humans, and foods—and by playing in the dirt as children. With changes in agricultural practices, modern diets that include a large percentage of processed foods, and the introduction of antibiotics, the need for supplementation is growing. But foods that support a healthy flora will provide your body with nutrients it understands how to utilize more fully. While a pill gives a controlled and measurable dosage, it's still limited to the strains that are easily procured and can be made shelf-stable. A variety of foods offers a wider

A variety of foods offers a wider array of beneficial microbes, and the more diverse the flora you take in, the healthier your immune system will be.

array of beneficial microbes, and the more diverse the flora you take in, the healthier your immune system will be.

Patients often ask if they can eat yogurt or other fermented foods in lieu of taking a probiotic during treatment. My answer is no—not while you are on antibiotics. It's important to take the higher-dose probiotic pills if you are on an antimicrobial regimen because the prescription and natural antibiotics will attack your beneficial gut flora as well as the microbes you want to get rid of. In addition to taking a probiotic, increase your intake of fermented foods such as yogurt, kefir, sauerkraut, miso, tempeh, kimchi, and kombucha. Even when your treatment is complete, continue eating these foods to enhance immune function; it's a beneficial lifelong habit.

Fiber, discussed above as a prebiotic, as well as those naturally occurring in fruits and vegetables, will help feed your beneficial bacteria by producing something called *short-chain fatty acids*. These create butyrates, which are food for the cells of the colon. The right balance of soluble and insoluble fiber is key. If your diet consists of mostly fruit, vegetables, and whole grains, and you have a moderate intake of animal protein and healthy fats, you are on the right track. If three-quarters of your plate or bowl is filled with plant-based foods and one-quarter is animal protein, you have an ideal ratio to support a healthy digestive system. For some, that amount of roughage may be too much for the gastrointestinal tract to handle; pulverizing vegetables and fruits in a blender and adding them to smoothies or pureed soups, or lightly steaming vegetables, can make them more digestible.

SUPPORTING BENEFICIAL YEAST BALANCE

Beneficial yeast is an important part of the microbiome, and it works in synergy with beneficial bacteria. When probiotic formulations are made with a blend of beneficial bacteria and beneficial yeast such as *Saccharomyces boulardii*, they have been found to improve treatment outcomes in cases of diarrhea or unhealthy colonization in the gastrointestinal tract.[6] Colonizing beneficial yeast is important to defend against pathogenic yeast cultures such as *Candida albicans*.

I want to touch briefly on a phrase used in the natural medicine world that patients often find confusing: I would like to step away from the phrase "systemic yeast overgrowth." A majority of yeast infections present in the body infect the surface only; even in the digestive tract or the vaginal canal, yeast are still on an external surface. The most common yeast pathogen is *C. albicans*, which adheres to tissues and triggers inflammation, causing fatigue, itching, gas and bloating, and changes in the skin and nails. This may also present as thrush (yeast overgrowth in the mouth), chronic vaginal yeast overgrowth, slow-growing patches on the skin, or red, moist lesions in the folds of the skin. Once the yeast attaches to tissue, it secretes enzymes that break down fats, cell membranes, and proteins.[7] This is probably why the term *systemic* is used, but the real problem is the buildup of systemic inflammation, not free-floating yeast molecules in the bloodstream.

In severely immunocompromised patients, colonization of yeast can happen in the organ systems; this is common in those who are suffering with HIV/AIDS, advanced diabetes, end-stage cancer, and other life-threatening illnesses. Typically, that sort of infection requires hospital-level care for candidemia (the presence of yeasts in the blood). *Cryptococcus neoformans*, a type of yeast, is commonly associated with life-threatening meningitis and can be drug-resistant to antifungals. However, this condition is rare.

The yeast infections I typically see are routine *Candida* overgrowth in the gastrointestinal tract, oral cavity, vaginal canal, skin, and nails. Many patients who present to my clinic with chronic Lyme disease have been ill for a long time and are already colonizing yeast; if this is the case, they are treated right away for overgrowth. The most common are chronic nail infections. However, once the internal yeast is balanced, the nails grow heathy again. It's very rare for patients with yeast overgrowth to get to the point that they require hospital-level care. In all my years of treating patients with antibiotics, I have never seen it. If a yeast overgrowth escalates and requires that high a level of care, a more serious illness is usually the underlying cause.

Those with chronic Lyme disease can have reduced immunity, allowing overgrowth of surface yeast, so it's important to evaluate for *Candida* with blood work before starting treatment, to avoid further complications. Blood tests for *C. albicans* are looking for antibodies that have been triggered by an immune response, due to exposure to nonbeneficial *C. albicans* in the gastrointestinal tract.

Treatment for yeast overgrowth depends on the severity of the infection. Natural yeast treatments are gentler and may be effective, but in some cases antifungal medications are the best course of action. Yeast can also create biofilms, which make an infection more difficult to treat. Most patients I see opt for natural treatments and make big changes in diet to correct the problem. This usually does the trick. Those who need more immediate care because of difficult symptoms can be treated with pharmaceuticals. This is a short-term solution offered with the idea that the patient will also make necessary changes such as reducing their intake of refined sugar.

Conventional medications aimed at eradicating pathogenic *Candida* are working to block the production of the vitamin D2 derivative Ergosterol. A study published in 2015 in the *Oxford Journal* found that supplementation with vitamin D3, which is more easily utilized in the human body than vitamin D2 (the plant form of vitamin D), was helpful in reducing the pro-inflammatory effects of *Candida* in mice. The study also found that people hospitalized for yeast infections of the blood were more likely to have low vitamin D levels. Based on this finding, you might think that higher doses of vitamin D would be helpful, but the research showed that a mild to moderate dose was a better option. Higher-potency dosing was actually counterproductive, supporting conditions ripe for yeast.[8] Unfortunately, the study did not give optimal dosing, which means there is still no clear consensus on dosing strategy.

EATING AN ANTI-YEAST DIET

The best way to keep yeast in balance—better than any supplement—is with diet. Treatment failure for yeast and for tick-borne disease is more likely if the patient continues to consume foods made with white flour, white sugar, and high-fructose corn syrup while they are being treated for a yeast infection. Botanicals with powerful antifungal properties are also an option. Beneficial microbes can crowd yeast out, so consider supplementing with *Saccharomyces boulardii*, a beneficial yeast. The other way to kill yeast is to stop feeding them. If you feed a seagull bread, twenty others will arrive wanting more. Yeast is like those gulls. It loves sugar, and the most delectable items to yeast are processed simple carbohydrates such as flour, processed sugars, and high-fructose corn syrup. If most of the food on your plate is white, beige, or brown, you are eating a yeast buffet.

Sugar is highly addictive, and eliminating it can cause an emotional reaction. I have seen many people become highly emotional—easily angered or saddened—after they've tried removing bread, pasta, and high-sugar foods from their diet. The body becomes accustomed to having a certain amount of sugar, and microbes want their fix as well. When you stop eating sugar, signals to the brain stimulate sugar cravings. As with cutting out any addictive substance, removing sugar from your diet could make you cranky, tired, or nauseous until your body recalibrates itself. On the flip side, when someone commits to making this change and is able to make it through the withdrawal symptoms, she experiences dramatic changes in her physical body. These changes include weight loss in individuals with a history of difficulty losing weight, healthy nails after long-term fungal infections, and improved digestive health.

I have found the Whole30 program highly effective for patients, and it offers a clear set of guidelines designed to reset the metabolism. Many program-specific recipes are available, which helps keep the diet more enjoyable—and that, in turn, helps people stick with it. The rules of the diet are commonsense ones: Avoid sweeteners, alcohol, grains, legumes, dairy, and food with preservatives. The best dietary goals are those changes you can sustain long enough to see positive change yet have a short enough time horizon that you can commit—thirty days is a good length. This is usually long enough to allow the sugar cravings to clear. Once you detox from sugar, the taste becomes too sweet and intolerable . . . imagine that! This is when you know you have kicked the sugar habit. Many of my patients choose to stay on the diet for longer periods of time, making it their daily eating plan.

One easy-to-find food that supports proper yeast balance is cold-pressed virgin coconut oil, which has a high concentration of caprylic acid, an antifungal. Ingest one to two tablespoons (14 to 28 g) per day at room temperature. Coconut oil can be taken on an ongoing basis. For a more potent effect, you can add one or two drops of oregano oil[9] or turmeric oil,[10] but do this only for one to two weeks. Ingesting essential oils can be therapeutic but is appropriate only for a short course of treatment; take the oils for no more than two weeks at a time, with extensive breaks in between. Be sure to consult with a practitioner trained in herbalism, aromatherapy, or the medical use of essential oils.

For a list of antifungal supplements to combat yeast overgrowth, together with dosing instructions, see the reference chart on page 232.

Implementing Detoxification in Daily Life

Toxins can create stagnation in the terrain of your body; just as the earth is the terrain you walk on, your body is the terrain you live within. We all see the effects of toxins and the overabundance of waste on the earth, but this also happens within the body, with the same ill effects. The body has a harder time clearing infections and toxins when it's overly burdened by toxins, stress hormones, infections, and unhealthy foods.

The ability of a person to clear toxins rests in genetics, lifestyle choices, emotional stress, level of infection, and continued exposure to external toxins. The good news is that we have the power to make changes and improve our health over time. Chronic illness can be disempowering, but it does not have to be. Making positive changes in your life is one area that you can control. Even one good habit can change whole pathways, especially those regarding detoxification, cellular growth, revitalization, epigenetics, weight loss, and pain. It takes patience to allow changes to manifest in the physical body if toxins have built up over years. This is where the commitment to daily positive choices is critical; only by repeating a good habit does it become just the way you live.

Your body is a highly intelligent, efficient vehicle with the ability to heal itself. This ability can be stifled, however, when an overabundance of toxins builds up. Here, I will try to narrow the wide topic of detoxification to the top priorities: These are the changes that will lead to a cleaner life. It may take some time to implement the changes and reap the rewards, but think of your improved lifestyle as a long-term solution—feeding your body with proper nutrition, practicing mindfulness techniques, and committing to exercise can turn on genes that bring you to optimal health.

IT'S NOT EASY BEING GREEN— BUT IT'S THE BEST COLOR TO BE

You can dramatically reduce your exposure to toxins by taking matters into your own hands and becoming more aware of green living. Take a moment and look under your kitchen sink. Do you see products that make you cough and your eyes water when you use them? Time to let them go because those chemicals are being absorbed by your lungs and are moving into your circulatory system. Look in your cabinets. Are you using nonstick cookware or microwavable plastics? Plastics can get into the food you eat and into your body, mimicking estrogens. Do you have a water filtration system? New parents strive to reduce chemical exposure for their babies, but why don't we continue to do this for ourselves as adults? Are we less precious? Following is a summary of ways to green your life:

- **Use green cleaning products.** Eliminate, where possible, common household chemicals such as cleansers, soaps, cosmetics, air fresheners, and dryer sheets or replace them with substitutes that are dye-free, biodegradable, and made from natural sources. Baking soda, vinegar, borax, and lemon juice can work well for surface cleaning. Or seek green-focused brands of cleansers and body soaps, now widely available in the marketplace.
- **Cook on the stovetop and in the oven, when possible.** Don't bake or cook using nonstick cookware. Instead, use stainless steel, glass, stoneware, ceramics, or cast-iron pans, when possible. Teflon flakes off into your food as you cook in these nonstick pans, and it also emits low levels of the toxin perfluorooctanoic acid (PFOA) as well as other plastics. Microwaving in plastic containers releases estrogen-like plastics into food, so avoid cooking or reheating food in plastic containers. PFOA is released over time and is retained in human tissues, increasing hormone-sensitive cancer risk as well.

- **Quit smoking.** You may feel that all the stress of treatment for tick-borne infection makes this is the worst time to quit, but there is never an easy time. Continuing to smoke while you are trying to recover from tick-borne disease prolongs the illness because toxins are coming in from the cigarettes, negating the work to treat the infections. This is true of e-cigarettes and vaping tobacco, too.
- **Consume clean, filtered water.** Drink plenty of filtered water, minimally sweetened with natural fruit juice if you need flavor. Water is our primary element for life, so plentiful, clean water is paramount to health.

Install a water filtration system if one is not already connected to your plumbing or your refrigerator. Many water filtration systems exist, and they vary in affordability and their ability to clear metal, microbes, chlorinated by-products, volatile organic compounds, and radioactive substances from the water (especially if you have well water). If an integrated system is outside your budget, there are inexpensive options such as pitchers that filter water and can be refilled and kept in the fridge.

You can have your water quality tested, which is especially important with well water. If you have been chronically ill since moving into a new residence, be sure to have your water professionally tested. Many patients are shocked to learn how many toxins are in the water in their home, and their health dramatically improves when the water issue is addressed.

- **Eat ethically raised, organic meat.** Be mindful of where your meat comes from and how it is raised and processed. Ideally, meat should have no added hormones or antibiotics. Livestock are fed antibiotics to counter the illnesses brought on by the large doses of hormones the animals are given to make them grow faster. Whenever possible, buy local through farm-share programs and be aware of whether the farm you purchase from adheres to humane practices. This is not just about the ethics of the company but about the quality of the meat. When animals are treated inhumanely, the fat content is unhealthy; animals under stress release stress hormones that are expressed in meat, which we then ingest.
- **Avoid genetically modified foods.** These are foods that have had their genetics modified in labs, with the idea of producing bigger yields, making the crops more resistant to insect infestation, and developing prettier fruit. However, the changes to the genes of the plants are altering the DNA of our gut flora and producing foods that do not give our bodies the same nutritional value.

Clean Eating: Get Savvy about Produce

Eat organic as much as you can afford to. Pay special attention to the fruits and vegetables that are least and most likely to have pesticide residue. Some vegetables and fruits are so saturated that no amount of washing will improve your toxic load. The list below, created annually by the Environmental Working Group, is an amazing resource for consumer rights helping identify the Clean Fifteen, those which are the least impacted by pesticide residue, and those which are heavily sprayed (the Dirty Dozen). You can get away with less concern buying conventional produce with the clean fifteen. Check the PLU number associated with the produce. The conventional produce with pesticides will be a four digit number from 3000 to 4000. The certified organic produce is a five-digit number starting with a 9. The genetically modified food is a five-digit number that starts with an 8. The list is updated periodically, so search online to confirm the most recent findings (Environmental Working Group [www.ewg.org]).

CLEAN FIFTEEN	DIRTY DOZEN
Least likely to have pesticide residue	Highly concentrated with pesticides
Sweet corn	Strawberries
Avocados	Spinach
Pineapples	Nectarines
Cabbage	Apples
Onions	Peaches
Frozen sweet peas	Celery
Papayas	Grapes
Asparagus	Pears
Mangoes	Cherries
Eggplant	Tomatoes
Honeydew	Sweet bell peppers
Kiwifruit	Potatoes
Cantaloupe	
Cauliflower	
Grapefruit	

Skin Brushing

The skin is the largest organ in the body, and it continuously breathes in and out like an external lung. Physical therapies such as saunas and dry skin brushing can help this organ detox more efficiently. You can easily find a skin brush in the bath and body section of any store. Before your shower in the morning, take a skin brush and make light to medium brush strokes starting at your feet and moving up to your torso; then brush from the tips of your fingers up your arms toward your chest. This sloughs off excess skin cells and makes respiration easier for the skin; it also detoxes by stimulating lymph fluid to remove wastes from the system. An abundance of lesions on the skin, such as acne, can be a sign that the skin is getting bogged down, trying detox beyond its ability.

- **Clear the air.** Air purifiers vary in their ability to filter airborne microbes and toxins, and the cost will reflect the ability of the system to remove microparticles from the air as well the noise level of the machine. Many options are available, but start by researching IQAir filtration systems; you can then compare what best works for your home and budget.
- **Remove electronics from your body and your nightstand.** Turn off your cell phone at night, and do not use it as an alarm clock. Electromagnetic waves, even the low-frequency ones emitted by cell phones, can cause changes to tissue function over time. Use the speaker phone feature to keep the phone away from your head. Do not wear the phone in your bra, front or back pockets around the pelvic region, or anywhere on your body for long periods of time. For the same reason that cells phones are problematic, remove wireless routers from your bedroom or areas where you spend a lot of time.

TAKE A DEEP BREATH AND CARRY ON

Our lungs eliminate excess carbon dioxide and hydrogens, which maintains pH balance in the blood. Other than our outer layer of skin, the respiratory tract represents our first lines of defense against toxins. Air quality is important, but so is the quality of our breathing. Many people (including me) have developed a habit of breathing in the upper aspects of our lungs instead of

> **The more deeply we breathe, the more we release wastes and reduce the toxic effects of stress on our bodies.**

deeply from the diaphragm. This can start due to stress and then become habitual; you may not even realize you're doing it. Shallower breaths restrict oxygen flow and release of toxins.

Breathing, fortunately, can be corrected with yoga training, mindfulness practices, meditation, and exercise. The more deeply we breathe, the more we release wastes and reduce the toxic effects of stress on our bodies. Oxygen therapies—including hyperbaric oxygen tanks, intravenous ozone, and oxygen delivered via nasal cannula through portable systems—are sometimes used as a form of treatment for tick-borne disease as well.

LOVE YOUR LIVER

The most important organs to support for detoxification are the liver and the digestive tract. The liver has the all-important role of distinguishing nutrients from toxins in the foods we ingest. It converts carbohydrates, fats, and sugars into useful forms of energy for the body, and it tags toxins to be eliminated. The liver is made up of hepatocytes, cells that have an amazing ability to regenerate and heal. In fact, you can remove a good portion of the liver and it has the capacity to grow back! As the liver tags toxins to leave the body, they are sent to the digestive tract and kidneys for removal.

Focus especially on enhancing detoxification of the digestive tract and liver by avoiding foods that trigger inflammation, hydrating properly with filtered water, moving your body with yoga and other exercise, and taking herbal supplements that expel toxins. Another option is to participate in routine fasts in the spring and fall. If you have no experience with fasting, make sure to do so with medical assistance. Fasting typically should not be considered during times of active treatment for tick-borne disease, as successful treatment requires food to support the absorption of medications.

One of the main treatment goals is to help the liver cells in moving toxins through movement of bile, which flows through the caverns between each liver cell and picks up debris to dump into the intestines for removal from the body. You can support your liver and digestive system with castor oil packs, bitter greens, coffee enemas, and herbal formulations. As a culture, we have lost our love for and tolerance of bitter tastes, since they cannot compete with the enjoyment that salty, sweet, umami (savory), and sour flavors bring us. Introduce bitters back into your diet with leafy greens such as dandelion, arugula, endive, radicchio, watercress, and mustard greens. The bitterness can be cut slightly by blanching the greens, or by adding spices or acid in form of vinegars or lemon juice.

An old formulation, used since the early 1700s in Europe, is Swedish Bitters, made up of seven ingredients: aloe, rhubarb, saffron, myrrh, gentian, zedoary, and agarikon.[11] Bitters improve neurological stimulation of the digestive tract and promote proper digestion and mechanical release of bile from the gallbladder.[12] They also can be used to treat other conditions of the intestines, including parasitic infections, fungal infections, water retention, and inflammation. The intensity of flavor varies depending on the bitter herb you use, and this intensity can determine the effectiveness in treating the complaint.[13] Consult with a practitioner trained in herbalism to understand the type of bitter that would be best for your constitution; because of their ability to stimulate digestion, bitters may not be the right choice if you have inflammation in the digestive tract, reflux, or ulcerations.

Dandelion, a potent bitter edible plant, is generally regarded as safe for most people, unless they are allergic to ragweed or daisies. Most people want to pull up dandelions when they see them in the yard, but it's becoming common to see these vitamin-packed greens and roots in bunches in the produce aisle. Dandelion is beneficial to our bodies because of its antiviral properties; it also improves fatigue, decreases inflammation,[14] purifies the blood, and has been shown to have healing effects, restoring the cellular function of diseased liver tissue.

Glutathione is an antioxidant made up of the proteins glutamine, glycine, and cysteine. An important detoxifier and immune modulator, glutathione is found in highest concentration in the liver. It neutralizes toxins in the human body, supports mitochondria that create cellular energy, maintains healthy vitamin C levels, and moves heavy metals, especially mercury, out of the soft tissue of the body.[15] This powerful antioxidant is depleted with continued exposure to toxins such as alcohol, medications, trauma, infections, and heavy metals. A deficiency of glutathione can increase toxins such as ammonia, which increases neuroinflammation.

Glutathione can be supplemented orally, nebulized into the lungs, and delivered intravenously. The preferred route is intravenous or nebulization, but the oral liposomal glutathiones are improving in their absorbability. This supplement is commonly used to mitigate neurological symptoms related to multiple sclerosis, Parkinson's disease, and heavy metal chelation, and to reduce the impact of the Herxheimer reaction.

Binders such as bentonite clay, activated charcoal, modified citrus pectin, aloe vera leaf, and psyllium husk absorb or grab on to toxins in the gastrointestinal tract so they are eliminated rather than absorbed, and these are commonly used in treatment to reduce toxins in the body. These usually come in a powder form—simply add one-quarter to one-half teaspoon to six to eight ounces (120 to 235 ml) of filtered water. Typically, this is followed with

Detoxification Potential of Coconut Oil

SUPPLEMENTING WITH VIRGIN COCONUT OIL has been shown to improve antioxidant potential by enhancing glutathione production and superoxide dismutase levels. Coconut oil has the ability to improve liver enzyme levels as well.[16] Readily available in grocery stores, coconut oil can be taken daily; one to two tablespoons (14 to 28 g) per day is the optimal dose, but start with one teaspoon and build toward the higher amounts. You can simply swallow a spoonful or you can add it to coffee or tea, stir it into oatmeal, or spoon it into yogurt. Coconut oil also ideal for cooking—it has a high smoke point, which means it can be heated to high temperatures without creating harmful trans fats.

A common Ayurvedic practice called *oil pulling* entails swishing coconut oil in the mouth for ten to fifteen minutes daily, which pulls toxins and has been shown in studies to improve oral health.

another glass of plain water. Binders are best taken at least one hour before or two hours after other medications because they are not selective in what they bind. This could lead to lower absorption of supplements and other medications, reducing efficacy.

For a list of supplements, see "Common Herbs and Nutrients Used for Detoxification Support" on page 224.

Supporting the Body with Antimicrobial Herbs

Plant-based medicine is not just about the chemical constituents of the plant—it's not like taking a prescription—it's about the vitality of the plant resonating with the needs of the human to heal. According to herbalist Matthew Wood in *The Book of Herbal Wisdom: Using Plants as Medicines*, we are inviting a "magical experience" when we work with plant medicine. Historically, shamans and herbalists have learned about the medicinal properties of plants by communicating in meditative states with the consciousness of the plant to learn how they can benefit humanity.

Plants inhabited the earth approximately five hundred million years ago, whereas the earliest human remains that have been found are approximately 2.8 million years old. Plants have a deeper relationship with the earth and have had more time to perfect their ability to survive. They have been our food, shelter, and medicine, and they maintain the air we breathe. Plants are at the roots of conventional pharmacology; many active ingredients synthesized in modern pharmaceuticals were originally isolated from plants. They are also conscious beings with the ability to communicate with one other, to learn, and to respond to our emotional cues.

Herbal antimicrobials can be just as aggressive as antibiotics and, like antibiotics, can produce a Herxheimer reaction. Many patients have learned this the hard way, underestimating the power of plants and thinking they would get through treatment faster if they took higher doses. Patients are often surprised at just how powerful the herbs can be. Once patients clear some of the infection from their body and build up strength, they may later use antibiotics as needed.

Herbal antimicrobials are the most frequently administered and asked about therapies in my office. Because of the persistence of *Borrelia burgdorferi* and other tick-borne infections, antimicrobials are important to the healing process. These can be used alone or in conjunction with antibiotics. Many patients elect to use only natural antimicrobials, based on their individual comfort level, belief system, and concerns about past adverse reactions to antibiotics. I always support this choice fully. In many cases, I also elect to start with herbal antimicrobials alone if the patient is too weak to handle antibiotics. Antibiotics many be added later if symptoms persist.

Typically, regimens consist of herbal tinctures; the concentrated liquid form makes it easier for a patient to find optimal dosing. Dosing depends on the herb and on the patient's specific needs. While many blends are commercially available, I also make specialty herbal blends in the office, as needed. For those patients apprehensive about experiencing a Herxheimer reaction, tinctures give more control; the dose can be modified up or down, depending on response. Patients start with one drop per day added to two to four ounces (60 to 120 ml) of water, and increase that by one drop every three to four days, as the patient can tolerate without experiencing symptoms flares. Some individuals are very sensitive to antimicrobials, and must start by adding one drop to two ounces (60 ml) of water but drinking only one ounce (28 ml) of the water, thus taking half a drop. Others may take only one drop every two or three days. For those who are really reactive, I suggest that they rub a drop into their skin or add a few drops to a bath. For most herbal antimicrobials, the maximum dose is thirty to forty drops per day in two to four ounces (60 to 120 ml) of water. Starting with one drop per day, it takes a long time to gradually work up to thirty drops per day.

The most common method of administration for herbal medications are liquid preparations in combination formulas; in these formulas, several plant extracts are mixed together for their synergistic and additive effect. Typically, when mixing herbal extracts on your own, choose three to five plants that will be beneficial, based on your treatment goals. If you do not feel comfortable mixing your own, please use them individually or consult a practitioner trained in herbalism. The following companies are those I use most often in my practice: Byron White Formulas, Beyond Balance, LymeCore Botanicals, Bio-Botanical Research, Herb Pharm, Nutramedix, Elk Mountain Herbs, Chinese Classics, Misty Meadows, Wise Woman Herbals, and Gaia Herbs.

A diversified antimicrobial protocol can increase the likelihood that the medications will get into hard-to-reach tissues and work with more than one organ system for a better outcome. Both natural and conventional antimicrobials have the capacity to create a healing crisis with a Herxheimer reaction. The main difference with herbal antimicrobials is that you have more control over the amount taken.

For a list of supplements used for antimicrobial purposes, see the chart "Antimicrobial Herbs" on page 225 and "Essential Oils with Antimicrobial Properties" on page 232 . The list of antimicrobial herbs is vast, and there are many options beyond the ones I've included, but those I list have been well documented for their antimicrobial properties. This list is meant as a reference; please contact a practitioner trained in herbal medicine to help find the best option for your needs and constitution. Natural medicine is not a one-size-fits-all process; instead, it's a wide open, creative experience with many options.

Biofilm Busters

The goal in reducing biofilm is to access the microbes within the biofilm and make antimicrobial medications more effective. Biofilm is built by bacteria to help them withstand host immunity and changes in pH, and to create for the bacteria an environment in the body that is hospitable to their survival.

It is best to take a biofilm-busting supplement on an empty stomach and to avoid eating for two hours after ingesting it, alternating two weeks on supplements and two weeks off. Start with a low dose of one capsule initially because gastrointestinal upset may occur due to several bacterial and fungal microbes that live within the digestive tract. Side effects such as bloating and diarrhea or constipation may occur as the microbiome rebalances. If a patient has a history of small intestinal bacterial overgrowth, taking biofilm busters may aggravate those symptoms if they are not resolved. Get advice from a medical practitioner before starting on a biofilm buster.

In *Combating Biofilms: Why Your Antibiotics and Antifungals Fail*, James Schaller, M.D., suggests that it would be therapeutically beneficial to combine more than one biofilm buster and pulse the dosing. It's difficult to ascertain dosages for this, as the data are all over the place in terms of whether a high dose or minimal dose is more effective; also, enzymes historically have different units for dosage, depending on the brand. Whichever supplement you purchase, follow the instructions on the bottle—most formulas suggest one to two capsules twice per day. If you are working with a natural medicine provider, review the formulation and dosing instructions.

For a list of supplements used to fight biofilm, see the chart "Biofilm-Inhibiting Herbs and Nutrients" in the reference section on page 227.

Supporting the Adrenal Glands

We live in bodies that still function as though it were thousands of years ago, with primitive mechanisms for adapting to stress. The fight-or-flight response is designed to help us get away from a life-threatening situation. Historically, we faced dangers such as being chased by wild animals, starving, contracting disease, and being exposed to extreme elements, and our defenses are calibrated to cope with those threats. Now, our defense mechanisms are commonly triggered by things such as noise pollution, financial stress, annoyances, trauma, and being overworked. The past wasn't easy living by any means, but in modern times we face a great deal more stimuli. We are plugged in to technology for most of our waking hours, have a faster pace of life, and pack more activities into a day—all this can drain energy from the adrenal glands.

The adrenal glands rest atop the kidneys and are responsible for many metabolic functions such as immunity, adaptation, regular sleep cycles, cardiovascular balance, digestive balance, and blood sugar regulation. The adrenals are made up of the outer cortex and inner medullary. The outer cortex is further divided into layers that produce aldosterone, cortisol, and dehydroepiandrosterone (DHEA). The adrenal hormone system is intimately entwined with the nervous system.

The adrenal glands are constantly communicating with the hypothalamus and pituitary gland in the brain to maintain hormone balance as changes in the outer environment affect the inner environment of the body. Think, for example, about driving a car. A lot of sensory data is coming in continuously when you are on the road, and as long as the drive is uneventful, you probably feel calm. Then a person cuts you off, and you are jolted out of autopilot into a state where you need to react quickly to stay safe. Adrenaline is expressed from the adrenals, enhancing vision, bringing more blood to your muscles, increasing respiration to get more oxygen to muscles, and increasing your heart rate. When the situation is over, you notice that it takes time to feel normal again. The ability to get back to baseline is different for every individual. A person with a healthy, minimally stressed pair of adrenal glands will return to baseline fairly quickly. A person suffering from an illness, or one with a high-stress personality or a history of trauma, will have a more difficult time recovering.

When the body is stressed due to internal or external demands (think of the traffic aggravation I mentioned above), the adrenal glands will respond based on chemical messages from the brain, depending on the psyche's interpretation of the stressor. This can be good stressor, such as a celebration, or a negative stressor, such as a fear response. Each one triggers a response from the adrenal glands, and this response helps maintain multitasking, sustained energy, and quick thinking.

As negative stressors are prolonged during chronic illness, the adrenals try to help us survive. Beneficial adrenal hormones such as cortisol and DHEA are reduced due to the adrenals' inability to express enough to keep up with demand. Cortisol and DHEA help reduce the negative effects of prolonged adrenaline release, causing inflammation and blood sugar dysregulation. When cortisol and DHEA are both low, the person has increased symptoms of chronic fatigue, pain, weight gain around the middle, poor wound healing, and irregular sleep patterns, often with feelings of exhaustion because of continued insomnia. He may also have a tendency toward low blood pressure due to improper sodium and potassium balance regulated by the adrenals.

Adrenal fatigue contributes to female hormone dysregulation due to low cortisol levels. These low levels force the body to borrow from progesterone stores to make more cortisol, leading to progesterone dysregulation. Progesterone deficiency leads to shorter female cycles and irregular bleeding patterns. For most Lyme disease patients, both women and men, progesterone, estrogen, DHEA, and testosterone levels should be checked. We all have the same hormones, though appropriate levels are gender specific. Most of my patients have some form of hormone dysregulation due to stress and prolonged illness.

Hormone levels can be corrected over time with medication and, ultimately, by resolving the source of stress. The hormone imbalance may have started at an early age as the glands were maturing; cortisol levels can even be disrupted during a stressful birth. Many patients have suffered a traumatic childhood event or were not given adequate nurturing in a stressful home environment. Correcting the hormone imbalance may require a combination of herbal remedies, bioidentical hormone replacement (if needed), mindfulness practices, and trauma work.

Every patient in my practice is evaluated for adrenal function, which can usually be determined based on history of illness, sleep schedule, energy level, and metabolism, as well as evaluation of sex hormones. Those with low adrenal function also tend to experience a pattern of sugar cravings or sleepiness in the afternoon, around 1 to 3 p.m., with a surge of energy at 5 to 6 p.m. It can easily be treated with herbal support, B vitamins, homeopathic remedies, DHEA supplementation, and regularity in sleep schedule. The adrenal glands crave regular schedules.

For additional information on supplements to support the adrenal glands, see the chart "Adrenal-Supportive Herbs and Nutrients" on page 227.

Supporting the Body with Natural Anti-inflammatories

Changing the course of inflammation in the body is one of the areas where natural medicine shines. Through dietary changes, herbal support, and supplementing heathy omega 3/6/9 anti-inflammatory oils (fish oil and borage oil, for example), inflammation can be reduced in the body, changing the pathways that cause pain and degeneration. Treatment of inflammation is about striking a balance between pro-inflammatory and anti-inflammatory pathways. Without inflammation, our bodies would not be able to heal properly, as inflammation helps protect the body, clear toxins, and kill invaders. However, chronic Lyme disease triggers inflammatory proteins to be expressed over and over again, which weakens tissues over time. It also creates chronic relapsing pain in multiple areas of the body.

The immune cells primarily responsible for inflammation are cytokines. Cytokines are produced by several immune cells in the body in response to stressors—those cytokines most frequently seen in Lyme disease are IL-6, IL-8, and TNF-α. Lyme disease spirochetes cross the blood-brain barrier, triggering cytokines and promoting inflammation. The presence of these proteins can trigger cells to attack myelin sheaths (the protective fatty layer around nerves) and also enhances oxidative damage, mitochondrial dysfunction, and antibodies that attack the neurological tissue.

Some cytokines are anti-inflammatory, but *Borrelia burgdorferi* suppresses this pathway in the body. The continuous triggering of pro-inflammatory

Mast Cell Activation Syndrome

MAST CELL ACTIVATION SYNDROME (MCAS) is a constellation of symptoms that present as hives, abdominal pain, flushing of the skin, numbness, tingling, cognitive disorders, and more severe manifestations such as anaphylactic reaction. Anaphylaxis can lead to low blood pressure and loss of consciousness. Reactions often necessitate a trip to the hospital for emergency intervention. MCAS can develop with or without tick-borne infection as a trigger and is confirmed with symptoms history, specific blood markers, and urine markers.

Mast cells are immune cells found throughout connective tissue in the body; they release histamine in response to stress, which creates inflammation and swelling in the area. Identifying the trigger can be difficult, which is very stressful for patients because the response can happen out of nowhere. The treatments for MCAS are similar to those for tick-borne infection and are designed to reduce inflammation and detoxify the system. MCAS is a complex condition that requires care from those trained to treat it.

cytokines can create autoimmune-like symptoms and elevate inflammation markers in the blood associated with autoimmune disease.

Even when infection is present, autoimmune disease can be triggered. As the body tries to manage the imbalance of pro-inflammatory cytokines and clear a hard-to-reach infection deep in the tissue, the body attacks itself. Self attacking self is the very definition of autoimmune activation.

Combatting Neuroinflammation and Providing Cognition Support

When Lyme disease colonizes multiple areas of the body simultaneously, including the brain, it creates inflammation that impairs memory, causes brain fog, and creates mood imbalances, which can lead to extreme changes in personality, altered speech, abnormal gait, sensory overload, and autonomic dysfunction. This colonization of Lyme disease in the brain can also cause a person to feel separate from himself, a phenomenon called *deperson-alization*, and it can inhibit activities of daily living, disrupt sleep patterns, and increase pain.

Note that this constellation of symptoms is based on the number of neurotoxins circulating in the brain and the activation of neuroglial cells, a large group of cells that surround neurons and "glue" everything together. Glial cells are free-floating cells in the central nervous system. In the brain, they monitor and react to changes in the brain environment, and their importance in brain healing and regeneration can't be understated. They maintain proper neurotransmission, energy metabolism in the brain, and overall brain balance, and they ensure the integrity of the blood-brain barrier.

In particular, brain microglia (a type of glial cell) are the primary immune defense in the brain. However, microglia that are continually in a state of overstimulation called *microglial activation* can, over time, become part of the problem rather than the solution. Microglia are important to synaptic pruning of unnecessary neurons, tissue repair, and the scavenging of plaques and microbes that can cause injury to the brain. They are responsive to inflammation, which can be caused by leftover fragments of *Borrelia burgdorferi* in the brain. This debris can be present after anti-infective treatments.

Interestingly, a 2018 study titled "Primary Human Microglia Are Phago-cytically Active and Respond to *Borrelia burgdorferi* with Upregulation of Chemokines and Cytokines," published in *Frontiers of Microbiology*, found that human microglial cells, which function to ingest harmful substances in the brain, only absorb *B. burgdorferi* fragments killed by antibiotics, not those that are living. The living microbes are out in plain sight, but microglial cells are not triggered to clear them out. Only when *B. burgdorferi* exists as leftover dead fragments do the cells react. Much more research is needed to understand this response fully.

Natural medications have been helpful in improving neurocognitive function. They can help balance neurofeedback pathways in the body, improve blood flow to the brain, and support proper gut health because of the gut-brain connection. The beneficial microbes living in our small and large intestine participate in the regulation of neurotransmitters—mainly serotonin and gamma-aminobutyric acid (GABA)—via a communication pathway that uses the vagus nerve. This pathway is the primary communication between the brain and the gut, also known as the *second brain*, or the *enteric nervous system*.

The vagus nerve governs the parasympathetic nervous system, which stimulates cellular repair by supporting proper sleep patterns, healthy digestion, adaptation to stress, and an overall sense of calm. When we are calm, we seem to go through life more comfortably. Unfortunately, we often spend far too much time triggering the opposing system, the sympathetic nervous system. This system stimulates the fight-or-flight response, which creates the burst of energy you need to get through stressful situations. If this response is triggered too much, though, it can degrade the body's immune system and cause more inflammation. One of the simplest—and cheapest— ways to support your vagus nerve is through meditation (we'll explore the vagus nerve and the nervous systems more in chapter 10, when I discuss living with chronic Lyme disease).

One of the major pathways altered by inflammation when Lyme spiro- chetes invade is the one that produces serotonin, referred to as the *kynurenine pathway*. Serotonin is the amino acid that improves mood, helps regulate sleep, and maintains energy, libido, and appetite—in fact, many antianxiety medica- tions and antidepressants attempt to make more serotonin available by blocking it from leaving the brain. A nonmedication option for maintaining a healthy balance of neurotransmitters is to feed the brain the amino acids it needs to make the neurotransmitters such as 5-HTP and L-tryptophan, which are precursors to serotonin.

N-methyl-D-aspartate (NMDA) receptors are triggered by glutamate. Glutamate is one of the most abundant neurotransmitters in the body, used to send signals from one nerve cell to the next. It is also extremely important in cellular repair, neuroplasticity, learning, and cognitive function. Injury to the brain in the form of acute trauma or chronic afflictions such as chronic Lyme disease makes it more difficult for glial cells to maintain the proper amount of glutamate in the brain, leading to overabundance.

As discussed previously, the biggest problem with having chronic Lyme disease is the perpetuation of inflammation cycles that age the body prema- turely. Over time, inflammation markers are released in response to the presence of spirochetes in the brain. This can cause memory loss, learning impairment, psychological imbalance, and eventually brain injury. The most common inflammatory protein responsible for toxicity in the brain is quino- linic acid, which builds up in the brain as a result of overactive glial cells. Elevated levels of quinolinic acid have been found in blood serum and cerebrospinal fluid of those confirmed with *B. burgdorferi*.[17]

Herbs that have been shown to reduce neuroinflammation include curcumin/turmeric, *Gastrodia*, ginseng, ginkgo, green tea extract, licorice root, and *Uncaria rhynchophylla*.[18] Preliminary research has also shown that supplementing with the serotonin precursors L-tryptophan and 5-HTP can reduce neuroinflammation. Gluten-containing foods, on the other hand, contribute to the abnormal stimulation of NMDA receptors, which can explain the brain fog people experience after eating a piece of bread. Serotonin depletion can lead to increased cravings for sweets. It's best to feed the brain in a way that creates healthy serotonin flow throughout the day and to

King, Prince, Pauper

WHEN YOUR SEROTONIN LEVELS ARE LOW, you may crave sugary, unhealthy carbohydrates such as cookies, cakes, and soda; but these foods will only set the stage for more inflammation, blood sugar imbalance, and growth of yeast in the system. Serotonin precursors have a natural rhythm—they are more heavily expressed later in the day, as they participate in the sleep cycle.

The best plan for supporting healthy serotonin levels is to eat meals in order of king, prince, and pauper: Make breakfast the largest meal of the day; eat a midsize meal lighter in protein in the middle of the day; and have the lightest meal—consisting mainly of complex carbohydrates such as vegetables and fruits, healthy grains (quinoa, wild rice), and a small amount of protein—at the end of the day. The standard American diet typically involves little or no breakfast because we are in a rush and a heavy, protein-dense meal at night because we are ravenous after a long day. Flipping this pattern can help reduce weight and improve mood balance throughout the day as we better align with our bodies' natural neurohormone cycles.

supplement with the serotonin precursors listed above. Other supportive choices are regular exercise, light therapies used for seasonal affective disorders, and a diet rich in eggs, chickpeas, raw cacao, chicken, turkey, salmon, beef, and nut butters.

As much as we might prefer to manage our bodies naturally, for mood imbalances that are severe or caused by overwhelming life stressors, prescription medications may be necessary. My advice is to stay open to all therapeutic options, including pharmaceuticals, as the situation demands. Unfortunately, some patients associate antianxiety medications with being mentally or emotionally weak, or they fear they will become reliant on the medication. These are valid concerns, but if you are experiencing intense anxiety or sleep deprivation due to neuroinflammation, the priority is to calm the nervous system so it can heal.

For a list of supplements and herbs used to fight inflammation, see the chart "Natural Anti-inflammatories for Brain and Body" on page 228. These supplements can be taken with food and with other medications, with the exception of the proteolytic enzymes, which are best taken on an empty stomach at least an hour before eating again. If these enzymes are taken with food, they will use their action to break down the food instead of being absorbed into the digestive lining for therapeutic benefit. Note that you do not need to buy all of these supplements individually. Many natural anti-inflammatories appear in combination products that simplify the process of incorporating the herbs into your treatment. Those anti-inflammatories that are cooking herbs, such as curcumin, can simply be used more liberally in foods for their benefits.

In Summary

If you have a primary care doctor or Lyme-literate physician who has provided prescription medications but offered limited guidance on natural medications to support the process, the supplements discussed in this chapter and listed in the reference section at the back of the book will provide you with much-needed information. If cost is an issue or if you find this list overwhelming, I recommend prioritizing a high-dose probiotic (no matter the antimicrobial protocol), a detoxification supplement, adrenal support, and herbal antimicrobials.

The quality of the supplement is very important. Let the buyer beware when it comes to websites with supplements from third-party sellers, for there is no guarantee the product is authentic or that it was not tampered with or stored improperly. These supplements are the foundation that support your health, so take the time to learn how they work and what they can do for you. Seek medical guidance to tailor the most efficient medication combination for your health goals.

CHAPTER 8

THE FOUNDATION IS STRONG— NOW SUPPORT THE INFRASTRUCTURE

The therapies discussed in this chapter can serve as robust support for the body throughout the healing process. While the treatments we talked about in the previous chapter help create a solid foundation for conquering tick-borne diseases, you need to do more than build a foundation—you need to support the infrastructure so that you have greater energy, mobility, and well-being, and stronger immunity. Here, you'll find simple, accessible options for doing that, from homeopathy to flower essences to essential oils—all of which support the mental, emotional, and physical body.

The Premise of Homeopathic Medicine

Outlined in the early nineteenth-century book *Organon of Medicine* by Samuel Hahnemann, M.D., homeopathy is a system of medicine based on the

Law of Similars. The premise is that giving small doses of a physical substance that causes symptoms in larger doses heals those same symptoms. In a homeopathic dilution, the substance can be mineral, plant, medication, animal, or microbe. Diluting the substance enhances the potency of the energies for healing purposes and avoids the negative effects of the physical substance. It provides the body with the information needed to change its circumstances. The medication delivered is in such small amounts that it's no longer physically present in the carrier substance (usually water, alcohol, or sugar pellets).

This was a difficult concept for me when I first started in my naturopathic doctorate program, but after studying the topic intensively for two years in medical school, relying on my own experience, and observing the amazing changes in patients over a decade, I have found homeopathy invaluable. While it may sound impossible for the dilution to be medically useful, homeopathy represents a form of quantum healing. The energetic imprint of the substance remains in the liquid dilution or pellets. This dilution primarily changes our water, a majority of our physical substance. You can get a better understanding of water's ability to change its form with new information by reading a book by Masaru Emoto, doctor of alternative medicine, such as *The Hidden Messages in Water* or *Love Thyself.*

Miasms

Dr. Hahnemann noticed that each patient presented with a particular constitution, temperament, physical characteristics, likes and dislikes, and family patterns, which he referred to as *miasms*. Miasms are imprints or tendencies within a person, and they create a predisposition to certain diseases. These are passed down through the generations in families. If a family was exposed to a certain disease during an epidemic, for example, that exposure could change genealogical history if not fully resolved with healing of the mind, body, or soul; this may manifest on an individual level as things you are attracted to or dislike.

Miasms may influence the environments in which you feel at peace or in conflict, your aversions and attractions, and the time of day you are most alert. If your tendencies create stress on your body and mind, your health can be affected. This can weaken your immune system, hormone system, and neurological system. Miasms can play a role in disease states and how you might manifest them. A unique constellation for every person, miasms are both conscious and unconscious.

We all have miasms on some level, but healing happens when we develop a deeper understanding of our inherited baggage and let it transform into new patterns, which can heal your current life as well as the lives of your descendants. If energy blockages, inner emotional conflicts, trauma, and unhealthy family patterns persist over time, however, they can cause disease states.

The amount of data collected and categorized in homeopathic references is immense, and a full exploration is beyond the scope of this book. This information has been collected over two centuries by many practitioners who witnessed consistent outcomes after dosing people with certain substances; they then documented the mental, emotional, and physical changes. My goal is to familiarize you with the concepts surrounding homeopathy, as the therapies are so widely available. A form of therapy rooted in individualized medicine, homeopathy is something I use daily in my practice to help patients in healing many conditions. I have found it can be implemented with other therapies, even conventional medications. I was trained in constitutional homeopathy. In this branch of homeopathy, we identify a specific remedy after taking a detailed patient history and comparing it with detailed data on remedies collected by practitioners for a few hundred years.

I frequently use homeopathic nosode therapy and homeopathic drainage. Homeopathic nosodes are highly diluted preparations of dead microbes such as the bacteria that cause tick-borne infections, viruses, parasites, or funguses. To be clear, there are no active infections in a nosode remedy; they are energetic imprints that provide the body with the information it needs to overcome symptoms. Homeopathic drainage uses combinations of minerals and botanicals to help with the clearing of toxins; these formulations, which are geared to specific organ systems, help patients regain healthy organ function and energy. Consult with a naturopathic doctor or practitioner with a professional certification in homeopathy to find the right formulation for your particular health condition.

Low-Dose Immunotherapy

Low-dose immunotherapy (LDI), developed by Ty Vincent, M.D., expanded on low-dose allergy therapy, which has been used for decades to expose the body to very low doses of a substance known to cause allergy, whether that is a food, medication, microbe, or an environmental factor. The therapy is intended to retrain the body to ignore these harmless substances. Dr. Vincent borrowed from this treatment concept, expanding it by using dilutions of infectious diseases, primarily tick-borne infections. The therapeutic value is in exposing the body to diluted amounts of infectious diseases, which changes the body's response to one of tolerance rather than of reaction. The microbial immunotherapy dilute is typically paired with the enzyme beta-glucuronidase, further enhancing the treatment's effectiveness in shifting the immune response. In my experience, the medications can also be effective without this added enzyme, which is the way I typically dose it in my office.

If tick-borne disease and other microbes can persist in the body even with treatment, then LDI offers an option that helps the body be at peace with the presence of the microbe. As I've discussed previously, the most problematic issue with Lyme disease, as well as other persistent microbes in the body, is triggering of the immune response, which creates persistent inflammation, causing tissue damage and suffering. LDI changes the behavior of the immune cells so they are no longer in attack mode. According to Dr. Vincent, LDI enhances the function of the T suppressor cells, which calms the response that leads to many autoimmune conditions. I have seen good results with LDI, leading to both immediate and continuous improvement as patients return for treatment at regular intervals. I have seen higher energy, reduced headaches, less ringing in the ears, lower light sensitivity, and decreased pain.

LDI remedies are created with dead microbes acquired from a specialty lab. No live infections are ever used. These dead microbes provide information in the same way that homeopathic remedies do, via leftover proteins, which are then diluted with sterile water. Through this process, solutions with different potencies are created from the mother tincture. These can be administered as a subcutaneous shot with a small bubble of liquid placed under the skin or sublingually (under the tongue) for those who prefer oral dosing to a shot. The immunotherapy shots are affordable compared with other therapies and require administration approximately every two months. LDI can be used as a primary therapy or in combination with other treatments.

As with any therapy, when the treatment works, it works well. While not everyone is responsive, I feel it's worth trying. The remedies have many different dilutions, so it's possible to tailor the specific dose to the individual. My interest in offering LDI as a treatment in my clinic was piqued because my primary patient population is infected with tick-borne disease and tends to be willing to try new therapies if they might enhance quality of life. I have seen symptoms improve, together with lab values that show a higher antibody level on the Western blot as well as the CD-57, in patients using only LDI. These positive outcomes depend on the individual's immune system, but LDI is a promising form of therapy for the rising number of people with chronic infections.

Flower Essences

Think about being near a flower, with its vivid color and sweet scent, and you can feel your mood lift. You are connecting with the essence of the plant using your sense organs, both your physical sense organs and subtle senses of intuition, to connect with the remedy. Flower essence remedies are based on formulations brought forward by Edward Bach, M.D., homeopath, bacteriologist, general family physician, and researcher in the 1930s. A very intuitive doctor, he connected the emotional imbalance in patients with an appropriate expression of support from the plant realm, specifically flowers. Dr. Bach started with a list of 38 remedies, and other practitioners have since expanded this list. As with homeopathy, the data have been collected by many practitioners over time, as they repeatedly observed patient outcomes. Flower essences can be researched further by visiting the websites of such organizations as the Bach Centre (www.bachcentre.com) and Green Hope Farms (www.greenhopeessences.com) or by reading one of the many books on the topic.

The flower essences support the emotional body through life challenges. Homeopathy works on the level of the physical body as well as the mental-emotional body. Homeopathic remedies are made in levels of varying potency, while flower essences imbue their energy signature into the water itself as the flower parts steep in water. Flower essences can be taken internally, applied externally, used in baths, or sprinkled on food. I recommend them frequently to help calm patients' anxieties, improve mood and sleep quality, and support them through emotional traumas. You can start by simply selecting a flower essence that corresponds to an issue you want to address and adding five drops of the essence to your water bottle, then drinking as you normally would throughout the day.

Electrolytes

As simple as it sounds, electrolytes offer great benefit to counter adrenal fatigue and autonomic dysfunction in those with chronic tick-borne infection. It's important to supplement with electrolytes when a person with tick-borne disease has symptoms of fatigue, postural orthostatic hypotension (a drop in blood pressure upon standing), lightheadedness, frequent fainting spells, persistent sweating, and muscle spasms. Chronic infections deplete the body of electrolytes, making it more difficult to maintain balanced hormones and neurological function and adapt to stressors, thus leading to symptoms associated with autonomic dysfunction.

Vitamin D Supplementation

VITAMIN D TESTING IS BECOMING MORE COMMON as part of routine annual blood work. Its clinical relevance and dosing have been underemphasized due to several decades of fear surrounding the toxic effects of vitamin D excess. In Great Britain after World War II, too much vitamin D was added to milk products, with ill effects on infants and toddlers. At that time, it was commonly added in large doses to milk and cereal and was even marketed as enhancing the health effects of beer because it was known to prevent rickets, a bone-weakening disorder that causes bowing of the legs, delayed growth, and body pain. These high doses created body pain, nausea, and vomiting, discovered to be due to vitamin D toxicity. The backlash led to the belief that anything more than what would be found in a tablespoon of cod liver oil—about 400–800 IU—could potentially be toxic.

Vitamin D is delivered primarily by ultraviolet light, when the skin is exposed to sunlight. It is then converted in the kidneys to its physiological form and helps in the absorption of key minerals for bone development.[1] Food sources of vitamin D include meat, fish, fortified foods, and cod liver oil.

It is important to supplement with the vitamin D3 form rather than the D2 form. The common prescription form of vitamin D is vitamin D2, the plant form, but the human body has to do further work to convert it to the animal form, D3. A typical dosage can range from 1,000 IU daily to 50,000 IU of vitamin D3 once weekly. Dosing is variable because of differing opinions among practitioners. The most common doses are 5,000 IU daily or 50,000 IU once a week. Proper dosing is dependent on whether vitamin D is being given for maintenance or to normalize dramatically low serum levels. The optimal level for this vitamin is 60–70 ng/ml; however, many Lyme disease patients suffer from low vitamin D, in the 30 ng/ml range.

The relationship of vitamin D deficiency and susceptibility to infection has been well documented for almost a century, but research shows that chronic bacterial infections can lower serum vitamin D levels by upregulating inflammation markers that downregulate vitamin D receptor genes.[2] Other viral infections can also lower vitamin D receptor activity, including Epstein-Barr[3] and *Mycobacterium* species.[4] To stay current on vitamin D research, visit the website of the Vitamin D Council (www.vitamindcouncil.org).

In those with chronic Lyme disease, the adrenals are low functioning, which is a problem because they manage the balance between sodium and potassium in the body. When electrolytes are depleted, the body has a difficult time with fluid balance, causing dehydration, cardiovascular instability, low blood pressure, muscle weakness, sleep disturbance, and neurological disruption. If you are tired and are drinking water but never feel hydrated, this could be an indication that you have adrenal fatigue leading to electrolyte imbalance.

Water follows the electrolytes in the body. When a person is trying to avoid heatstroke in intense heat, he will often take salt tablets (sodium is an electrolyte) to help hold in water. Lowering salt intake, on the other hand, can reduce water retention. Proper water and mineral balance are important to our daily functioning.

To add electrolytes, you can stir electrolyte powder into water (follow package instructions) and consume it throughout the day, or you can drink one of the many prepared waters infused with electrolyte supplements. I caution against using conventional replenishment drinks that have high sugar content and are colored with dyes. If you are blasting your hormone system with sugar and chemicals, you are defeating the purpose of adding electrolytes, which is elevating health. Keep your electrolyte products simple and choose those with minimal ingredients beyond the minerals themselves. This is true for any supplement purchased in the marketplace. If the "other ingredients" list on the bottle shows more ingredients than are on the minerals list, put the supplement back on the shelf.

Intravenous (IV) Therapy

In medical school, my primary focus was training in the use of intravenous (IV) therapy, and I concentrated on environmental medicine, the study of toxic burden on the body and of how to relieve this burden so the body can return to healthy function. I was also interested in the immune-enhancing ability that IV therapy could deliver to support the body's fight against cancer and infections. IV therapy is administration of liquid substances—vitamins, minerals, chelation agents, amino acids, or electrolytes—directly into a vein.

IV therapy can allow a substance into the body at therapeutic doses that could not be taken orally. For instance, vitamin C (ascorbic acid) can only be ingested at doses of perhaps 3–4 g orally before the digestive system decides that's enough and the rest is eliminated; at these lower levels, vitamin C is an antioxidant, reducing the cellular damage from toxins and enhancing immune function. When used intravenously, vitamin C can be taken in amounts of 50–60 g, at which point it becomes pro-oxidative in a way that is helpful for fighting infection and cancer. At this dose, vitamin C increases the body's production of hydrogen peroxide, which is its method of killing bacteria, funguses, and abnormal cells.

IV therapy has also been useful in cases where digestive problems lead to malabsorption of nutrients, in infections such as mononucleosis, and as a means of detoxing harmful substances from the body. The most common IV treatments I use are vitamin/mineral combinations, chelation agents (ethylenediaminetetraacetic acid [EDTA], dimercaptosuccinic acid [DMPS]), glutathione, high-dose vitamin C, and hydration. These work beautifully as a stand-alone therapy for acute conditions or as an adjunct therapy in case of chronic illness.

Pain Relief

Pain management is at a critical place right now, due in part to the opioid crisis. The health care system is trying to discourage use of pain medications that may spiral out of control and help those who are taking pain control medications in a destructive way while at the same time providing robust pain management to individuals who truly need it. With tick-borne disease treatment, pain is one of the most common complaints, but it is difficult to address. Far too often, chronic Lyme disease patients who have debilitating nerve, joint, and muscle pain are denied treatment for pain because the seriousness of the chronic disease is not acknowledged.

Leaving people in chronic pain creates trauma and desperation and often leads patients to self-medicate, sometimes in harmful ways. They may obtain addictive substances illegally and potentially abuse these drugs, which only creates another illness to recover from. Many patients have reported using excessive amounts of alcohol, high-dose anti-inflammatories, sleeping pills, and illicit drugs just to find relief. Most had asked their doctor for help and been turned away. Unresolved debilitating pain is one reason patients with tick-borne disease make frequent trips to the emergency room.

Pain management is a complex topic because so many variables contribute to the experience of pain. Many techniques can reduce pain through mindfulness exercises and the therapeutic application of acupuncture. In addition, medicinal herbs such as cannabis—now legal in some states—offer a safer alternative for those whose pain remains at high levels. States where cannabis is decriminalized are also experiencing decreasing opioid use. I have seen a huge difference in patients who are able to use cannabis without fear of legal penalties. They report reduced use of NSAIDs, sleeping pills, and antianxiety medications, as well as improved well-being. As patients feel more stable, resume quality sleep, and reduce their pain levels, they are able to be more compliant with their medication regimen and recover with greater efficiency. Eventually, they are weaned from medications and are able to live their lives free of pain.

Cannabis

CANNABIDIOL (CBD), DERIVED FROM *CANNABIS SATIVA,* is a nonpsychoactive constituent of the plant (tetrahydrocannabinol [THC] is the psychoactive constituent). CBD and THC are similar in molecular configuration but act very differently. The reason we humans react as we do to cannabis is that we already make our own cannabinoids through the endocannabinoid system, which acts in many different tissues in the body to maintain balance immunologically and neurologically.

THC has been indicated for reducing nerve pain, reducing muscle spasticity, improving cognition and digestion, and reducing anxiety. It modifies inflammation by activating CB2 receptors on immune cells. CBD is thought to subdue or block the response of cannabinoid receptors in our brains—specifically CB1, where it does not actually fit into a receptor but links to the side of the protein to decrease the function of the receptor. The fact that it does not go directly into the receptor, as THC does, is the reason CBD products do not produce a high. CBD also has a higher affinity for CB1 receptors in the neurons, which is why CBD offers greater benefit for seizure-like activity. CB1 receptors are found primarily in the nervous system, whereas CB2 receptors are linked with the immune system.

CBD and THC, when ingested, lose a lot of their potency through the digestive process—on average, only 6 percent is bioavailable.[5] These products are available in many forms, including as oil, capsules, dried (for smoking), and made into edibles such as chocolate squares and gummies. The most common options among my patients are oil blends and gummies. I can legally only dispense CBD. THC products are regulated by formal dispensaries across the country, depending on state laws. Dosing is difficult to discuss because there are so many different formulations, plant species (*Cannabis sativa, Cannabis indica, Cannabis ruderalis*), and patient-specific needs. Talk with your medical provider if you are looking to integrate cannabis into your treatment plan so you can find the best combination and dosage for your needs.

Mitochondrial Support

Mitochondria are the power generators of the cell. If mitochondria are not in good health, it is difficult for the body to remain well. A unique aspect of our physiology, mitochondria developed a symbiotic relationship within the human body; they are actually distinct living entities. While they did not originate from us, over millions of years mitochondria have become a part of us. All cells have varying levels of mitochondria within them, depending on their function and energy needs. Their primary role is to make adenosine triphosphate (ATP), which functions as our cells' fuel.

Like other parts of the human body, mitochondria can get overwhelmed with infections and toxins, which reduces their energy output.

Like other parts of the human body, mitochondria can get overwhelmed with infections and toxins, which reduces their energy output. As this happens on a wider scale with systemic illness, cellular repair mechanisms and energy are depleted and the aging process is accelerated. Mitochondrial dysfunction can be either genetic or acquired through diseases that affect organ systems, including the cardiovascular, neurological, musculoskeletal, and digestive systems. Most individuals with mitochondrial dysfunction are affected by acquired dysfunction. The good news is that, with detoxification and proper nutrients, mitochondria can recover.

I also suggest having a "dialogue" with mitochondria, visualizing them as strong, healthy, and restored. This is best done during meditation or before you take a supportive supplement. The body and its inhabitants are highly responsive to intention. Supportive nutrients that feed your mitochondria include:[6]

- **Alpha lipoic acid:** Antioxidant, anti-inflammatory, detoxifies mitochondria, reduces cytokines, and enhances glutathione. *Dosing is commonly 200–600 mg daily.*
- **L-carnitine:** Helps transport healthy fatty acids into the cellular membrane for proper function. Affinity for cardiovascular cells, antiaging support, and energy enhancement. *Dosing up to 2,000 mg per day shown safe.*
- **CoQ10:** Antioxidant, especially with oxidative damage of the neurological system. Upregulates gene sequences for metabolism and detoxification. Depleted with statin medications. Improves endurance. *Dosing up to 1,200 mg per day.*
- **NADH/NAD+:** Improves cognitive dysfunction found in neurodegenerative disorders. Improves chronic fatigue. Improves attention. *Dosing can be 5–20 mg; there are also nasal sprays available on the market for enhanced absorption.*
- **Membrane phospholipids:** Replace damaged mitochondrial membranes. Symptoms improved associated with chronic fatigue and fibromyalgia. *Dosage varies depending on product. Can come in powdered, liquid, or capsule.*

Essential Oils

In terms of treatments that are easy to find, are simple to apply, and yield real results, essential oils make the grade. For tick-borne disease, essential oils can act as antimicrobials, reduce stress, support a healthy immune system, and reduce symptoms associated with inflammation, including pain. They are also very helpful during minor acute illnesses such as upper respiratory infections and can serve as antiseptics for minor wounds.

The impact of essential oils on emotions is also well established, and they can be helpful in calming people with issues such as post-traumatic stress disorder and other stress-related conditions. In one study, lavender infused into the air of a designated nursing area of a trauma intensive care unit was shown to reduce stress among the nurses, potentially leading to improved retention and job satisfaction.[7]

The journal *Frontiers in Medicine* published a study that looked at 34 popular essential oils and their effects on *Borrelia burgdorferi* in the petri dish. Researchers found that oregano, clove bud, and cinnamon bark offered the greatest antimicrobial effects against *B. burgdorferi* and hindered biofilm formation at the lowest concentration. Oregano oil has the most potent effect, due to its active ingredient, carvacrol, which works to hinder both spirochete growth and biofilm formation. Bergamot has also shown great promise in inhibiting spirochete growth.[8]

Essential oils can be used in blends or individually. Eucalyptus, for example, can be mixed with myrrh to reduce inflammation and act as an antimicrobial. Add a little clove to combat throbbing sensations and add chamomile for a calming effect and to reduce nerve pain. Essential oils can be added to baths, applied topically with proper dilution, expressed into the air with diffusers, or used in massage therapy and Reiki sessions to enhance the therapeutic experience.

When deciding on an essential oil, note that not all oils are free of toxins—chemicals may be used to extract the oils from plants, and these chemicals are retained in the oils you are applying to your skin or, potentially, ingesting. Quality is important; not all oils are created equal. When choosing a supplier, make sure the company uses pure, organic botanicals and that it employs regular testing to ensure it is meeting quality standards. There will be some natural variability of the active ingredients in the oils, depending on the location where the plants were harvested and on the weather conditions the season they were grown.

While it has become popular to ingest oils for daily health maintenance, this is not historically how they were used. When I studied medicine, I was trained in the use of essential oils. They should only be ingested short term and should be managed by a provider with extensive training with herbal medications and aromatherapy. Peppermint oil, as one example, should not be consumed on a daily basis, as recommended by some, because the oil disturbs microflora, data on the long-term effects for internal use are limited, and it can be irritating to the sensitive tissues of the digestive tract. The essential oil is very different from a breath mint!

Essential oils can be administered in the following ways:

- **Topically:** Oils used topically should be mixed with a carrier oil, such as sweet almond oil or olive oil. You can keep the mix in a small bottle with a dropper or in a roll-on bottle. Apply the oils, as needed, to the affected area, such as an area of tension on the neck. Before using on a larger surface area of the body, perform a spot test by rubbing oil onto a small area of the arm and waiting an hour to check for a reaction. Some oils, such as citrus and bergamot, can cause photosensitivity or skin irritation. Oils can also be added to an Epsom salt bath for pain relief—it only takes a few drops.

  The dilutions below are typically added to a carrier oil such as almond oil, olive oil, or castor oil and used topically. Just about any oil is safe to use as a carrier for external application.

Percent Dilution	Drops per 1 oz (30 ml)	Use
2 percent dilution	10–12	Aromatherapy
3 percent dilution	15–18	For pain
25 percent dilution	125	Super strength

- **Aromatically:** Oils placed in a diffuser can spread their antimicrobial effects over a large area. Diffusing antibacterial and antiviral oils throughout the house is especially helpful during cold and flu season. Adding a few drops of oils to a facial steam bath can kick out a sinus infection very effectively. Diffusion can balance moods such as depression or anxiety as well. When oils are inhaled, they go straight to the areas of the brain that control emotions.

- **Internally:** I do not suggest internal use of essential oils on a regular basis, but in some circumstances taking oils orally can be useful. Black cumin seed oil and oregano oil are both useful anti-inflammatories that can be taken internally for short periods of time under the guidance of a trained practitioner.

For further study of essential oils, refer to *The Complete Book of Essential Oils and Aromatherapy* by Valerie Ann Worwood or *Releasing Emotional Patterns with Essential Oils*, 2018 edition, by Carolyn L. Mein, D.C. Avoid references written by essential oil companies, as the information may be skewed. Once you have your reference and your oils, have fun! Get to know them, and see how they make you feel. Generally, if it makes you feel good, it's an oil your body wants. If the oil stops smelling good to you, that may be an indication it's no longer needed. Each of the oils has a different personality, and the more you use them, the more familiar you will become with their properties.

For more information on therapeutic essential oils, see the chart "Essential Oils with Antimicrobial Properties" on page 232.

In Summary

These natural remedies can all be integrated into your treatment protocol for tick-borne disease, and you should investigate and experiment to see which ones resonate with you. Homeopathy and flower essences are best used with assistance from a medical practitioner because we are not always able to see ourselves or those we love clearly when it comes to self-prescribing. Supplements recommended for mitochondrial support are easily acquired and simple to use: Just follow the recommended dosing instructions on the packaging.

The use of cannabis for pain management does require assistance, in my opinion, to assess the appropriate brands, strengths, and THC/CBD combinations, and for advice on how to implement it for the best outcome. You may get lucky and find the perfect dose for you, but most patients who buy CBD oil on their own get poor results and then abandon it altogether.

Just knowing these treatments are available options is enough to get you discussing them with your medical practitioners. For more detailed data, visit the reference guide at the end of this book.

CHAPTER 9

BUILDING YOUR FUTURE BODY: PHYSICAL MEDICINE

P hysical medicine uses movement, mechanical stimulation, heat, manipulation, and/or electrical stimulation instead of medications to heal the physical body. These techniques enhance strength, improve neuroplasticity, and mechanically move bacteria out of hiding with improved circulation. This is why physical medicine is important to the treatment of chronic Lyme disease, no matter how minimal the approach. When we are inactive due to fatigue, pain, instability, vertigo, and/or depression, we can age prematurely, and this leads to a reduction in flexibility and fluidity and thus a lower quality of life.

Many patients come to the clinic after years of chronic illness and immobility. They frequently complain of a lack of flexibility and increased cracking sounds in their joints. Recovery requires reinforcing strength in the body. Think of it as building the body of the future by changing from the inside out and the outside in. One of my professors in medical school, Dickson Thom, D.D.S., N.D., used to say it took three to five years to fully change a human body—that is the time it takes to heal completely and reverse tissue damage. I feel this is also the time it takes to rewire the mind and to see the changes in the mind create changes in the tissue. Healing can be immediate, but realistically, we need to incorporate particular habits of movement, eating, thinking, and breathing to regain and maintain the health we seek. The energy propelling this will be willpower, intention, and hope.

Treatments will have different outcomes, depending on an individual's genetics, temperament, lifestyle choices, and health status. Our bodies are beautiful vehicles that give us the opportunity to move about the earth, interact with others, and accomplish tasks that give meaning to our lives.

Even with limitations, being at peace with our body and in healthy relationship to it is a critical part of getting well.

Sometimes, the body may want to just sit and be still, which is important too; but the ability to move our bodies freely and with vigor is one of our greatest gifts. Even with limitations, being at peace with our body and in healthy relationship to it is a critical part of getting well.

This chapter addresses the importance of physical medicine modalities that can support restoration as you recover. I am not trained in the use of acupuncture, massage therapy, or craniosacral work, but I'm discussing them here because I know they are valuable methods with plenty of data and positive patient outcomes to support their validity. Naturopathic doctors are trained in making adjustments to the musculoskeletal system, just as chiropractors and osteopathic practitioners are, as part of the degree program. Some choose to make this the focal point of their practice, while others home in on other specialties. Naturopathic doctors are also trained in minor surgery, but many practitioners are unable to perform procedures, depending on whether the state in which they practice allows minor surgery as part of the scope of practice. The same is true for chiropractic adjustment.

Physical medicine is not just about exercise therapeutics; it encompasses mechanical support for alignment of bones, muscle flexibility, and reduction in localized areas of pain, as well as subtler options such as craniosacral work. Exercise in some form is necessary if your recovery is to be wholly successful; it also reduces the amount of physical therapy you require after you have your strength back. Many patients lose confidence that their bodies will be able to do what they want them to do or they experience negative consequences, such as debilitating fatigue, after exercise. Some patients who exercise during recovery have increased Herxheimer reactions, and this can be a deterrent to further exercise.

Chronic Lyme disease can change the consistency and production of collagen fibers, which can alter the healing process of connective tissue—muscles, fascia, tendons, and ligaments. The presence of spirochetes and other tick-borne infections cause inflammation, altering the balance of hyaluronic acid (which lubricates tissues) and ground substance (a gel-like substance in extracellular spaces), and this changes the process of wound healing.[1] Acute injury and inflammation initially swell tissue, and chronic inflammation over time can atrophy or dry out ligaments, joint capsules, and other connective tissues, creating reduced mobility, weakness, and pain. Exercise, even light movement, lubricates and hydrates tissues, bringing in more nutrients while removing toxins. Supplementing with collagen type I/III or bone broth with also support healthy ligaments, tendons, and joint capsules.

All physical modalities can bring greater awareness of the places we are holding on to tension in our bodies, create consciousness of the emotions needed to release this tension, and remove hindrances in the body that are causing discomfort. For maximum benefit, find an activity or treatment modality that attracts you, one that draws you to receive the therapy. Have realistic goals and work from a place of detachment, remaining open to whatever changes begin to happen. Your therapy may transform you in amazing ways you would not expect, but you could miss these marvelous effects if you are looking for a different outcome.

Exercise and Physical Therapy

One of the most frequent questions I am asked is whether I recommend exercise to Lyme disease patients. I have heard many different opinions on this matter from other practitioners, and my answer is that recovery is an individual process and that patients must be evaluated on a case-by-case basis to determine how much exercise they can accommodate while recovering. It depends, in part, on what the person was doing before he got sick.

If you are used to running marathons and have the endurance to run ten miles per day, you may need to scale back to five miles per day or less. If you were never one to exercise, this is not the time to start training for a triathlon. That may seem to be common sense, but I've had patients who wanted to show that Lyme disease was not going to get the better of them, and they chose to start a new intense workout regimen with an unrealistic fitness goal. When they can't accomplish it, they end up in bed, hurting and demoralized.

Being sick with a chronic disease requires that you tune in to yourself and know your limits. But it is not an excuse to avoid life. You may need to modify your normal pursuits for a period of time, but do your best to engage daily in something active. Make sure it is an activity you enjoy, to remind yourself that you are not your diagnosis. If you get stuck in the story of your limitations, they can become a self-fulfilling prophecy. This is a delicate balance of listening to your body while also pushing it to maintain endurance and strength. Start small, keep showing up, and give your body time to heal. Moderation is the healthiest option in just about every situation.

BUT FIRST, YOGA

Yoga in the form of yin yoga, yoga nidra, or restorative yoga is an easy place to start with exercise—these types are all about going inward. Yoga nidra is done while lying on the floor in a pose referred to as the corpse pose while being led through guided meditation to release tension held in the body. Yin yoga incorporates postures with fluidity and no expectation of precision, with postures held for gradually longer periods of time. Its primary focus is to go inward and indulge in the stretch, being as fluid as you wish and learning to allow the muscle to relax.

Yoga is essentially a system of balancing the breath and the posture to lengthen and strengthen the body, over time opening the flow of energy through breathwork and inviting the muscles to respond by becoming more relaxed. Through regular practice, you can become stronger within your core muscles or the postural muscle groups deeper in the body. There is also the enormous benefit of improved diaphragmatic breathing and quieting of the mind through meditative movement. Yoga studios will have a variety of practices, with Hatha yoga seeming to be the most accessible. Yoga was originally meant to enhance the ability of a spiritual initiate to sit comfortably and meditate for several hours. Over time, it has become a daily practice that keeps a person connected to self and helps the body stay flexible through the aging process. Yoga has also been used to reach higher states of bliss through controlled breathing techniques and movements, such as those practiced in Kundalini yoga.

MOVEMENT, RESISTANCE TRAINING, AND WEIGHT-BEARING EXERCISE

The most important part of any physical modality is discipline. Your chief responsibility is to keep showing up to your own daily regimen and to see your physical medicine practitioners, if that is something you can afford and integrate into your life. Many patients end up debilitated to the point that they are unable to drive, which makes it difficult for them to get to medical visits on a regular basis. Lyme disease symptoms that change from day to day, or even from moment to moment, also make integrating activity into daily life complicated. The goal is to integrate some kind of movement, even if that means beginning with simple exercise at home. Start with five to ten minutes per day and build over time—keep showing up for yourself. Go outside for a short walk; exercise your lower or upper body while lying on the floor or sitting in a chair if

Exercise is not just about the physical movement; it's about empowerment and motivation. It creates optimism and uplifts mood.

you feel standing is not safe. Even integrating a habit of stretching in bed, if that is all you can do, will help you maintain some flexibility. But exercise is not just about the physical movement; it's about empowerment and motivation. It creates optimism and uplifts mood. I also suggest some form of massage, physical therapy, and/or chiropractic care at least twice per month. For the best outcome, add these modes of therapy to your daily exercise routine.

A study published in 2015 in *Medicine and Science in Sports and Exercise* looked at the effects of resistance training on patients suffering from chronic Lyme disease and found that, after a routine of three sessions per week for four weeks, patients reported improved energy levels and showed measurable improvement with exercise performance. The specific exercises were primarily varying repetitions of the leg press, seated row, vertical chest press, standing heel raise, and supine abdominal crunch.[2]

Weight-bearing exercise, accomplished by strapping on wrist or ankle weights and walking around the house performing normal activities, can add muscle mass. Typical weights for this type of exercise are one to three pounds (455 g to 1.4 kg). You can also lift weights using low-impact handheld weights in the one- to five-pound range (455 g to 2.3 kg). After several repetitions, that one-pound (455 g) weight can feel like a brick. Repeat your exercises until you feel a slight burn and shake in the muscle. This should be slightly uncomfortable, like you are working the muscle, but you should not feel intense pain. Please stop if you experience serious discomfort or pain. Work with your doctor and physical therapist to create a regimen that is appropriate for your health limitations. The idea is to increase your strength and ultimately overcome those limitations.

QIGONG AND TAI CHI

Qigong and Tai Chi are gentle meditative modalities that have been clinically shown to reduce pain, are safe in their application, and are benign in their slow, controlled movements. Qigong dates back more than 5,000 years; though it is a movement modality, it is also related to Traditional Chinese Medicine, which I will discuss in the next section. *Qi* (Chi) means "vital energy for the body," and *gong* refers to a disciplined practice to achieve a higher level of skill. Tai Chi was initially designed as a tool of defense in martial arts, but it has also long been practiced for health effects, as it focuses on relieving the physical impact of stress.

Both these forms of movement calm the nervous system by blending movement, breathing, and meditation into a form of self-care, and both are

Stepping Up to Support Those with Chronic Lyme Disease: The Dean Center

IN NEW ENGLAND, WHERE MY PRACTICE IS LOCATED, a prestigious state-of-the-art institution opened its doors to chronic Lyme disease patients, exhibiting an attitude of nonjudgment and acceptance. The Dean Center for Tick Borne Illness within Spaulding Rehabilitation Hospital, right in Boston, was the first major institution for patients with tick-borne infection that provided much-needed physical rehabilitation services and sought to learn about the disease with the goal of changing the current medical model. Headed by David Crandell, M.D., and Nevena Zubcevik, D.O., this department has been critical for the morale of Lyme disease patients, who finally have acknowledgment and a place to receive care. The facility is designed to serve a population who require medically managed physical support to return to active and productive lives. This is a facility to keep an eye on as it collects and analyzes data that could change views of tick-borne disease from the inside out.

used to achieve optimal health and longevity. Movements are gentle and slow, allowing anyone to participate. The more consistent you are with the practice, the more aware you become of your own flow of energy and the relationship of energy flowing through the natural world.

Over the centuries, many teachers have developed styles of Qigong and Tai Chi practice, with movements related to those witnessed in the plant and animal realm. These practitioners used movement for personal healing, to harness healing energy so they can be of service to others, to achieve spiritual enlightenment, to expand the strength potential of the body, and to manipulate subtle forces related to physical matter, which can look like magic to the outward observer.

My personal experience is with Yi Ren Qigong, which I studied with Guan-Cheng Sun, Ph.D., founder of the Institute of Qigong and Integrative Medicine based in Washington State. Learning Qigong was so important in my awareness of the relationship between mind, body, and spirit throughout my healing journey; I use it regularly.

I commonly recommend Tai Chi and Qigong to my patients. Teachers of Tai Chi are easy to find, but, depending on where you live, you might find it more challenging to locate a Qigong practitioner. If you have access to a teacher, all the better, but videos that introduce the practices are readily available online.

As a medical practitioner, I feel safe advising patients to take up an activity of slow and controlled movements that have little chance of causing injury. My goal for my patients is to improve strength, body awareness, stability on their feet, confidence in their physical ability, and gait. These benefits are especially helpful for those who use walkers or canes for assistance. Devoting ten minutes up to an hour a day can benefit you by increasing your confidence in your physical strength, decreasing your stress and pain, and attuning you to your inner awareness (intuition).

As integrative medicine becomes more accepted, additional research will start popping up to validate its place in the healing arts. Qigong and Tai Chi have been the subject of several research studies tracking their power to improve quality of life, strength, and well-being. A study published in 2010 by the *American Journal of Health Promotion* found improvement in those practicing regular Qigong with regard to their cardiovascular health, bone density, physical functioning, steadiness on the feet, self-efficacy, and quality of life.[3] Bone density is usually increased through weight-bearing exercise; however, Qigong is minimally weight bearing. Nonetheless, the patient demographic of postmenopausal women showed an increase in bone density and lower rate of fractures in those practicing Qigong regularly. Cardiopulmonary function improved, high blood pressure dropped, and they improved endurance with exercise. They also functioned better physically, experiencing reduced pain and improved gait.

Healing with Chinese Medicine

I'm not formally trained in acupuncture, cupping, or moxibustion, so I can't speak from a place of authority on the subject. However, I have worked closely with acupuncturists in clinical practice, taken classes introducing Chinese medicine concepts, received many treatments over the years, and witnessed amazing outcomes with patients. I could not include a chapter on physical medicine modalities without mentioning the elegant systems associated with traditional Chinese medicine. It has been so important in my own healing journey through Lyme disease, pregnancy, and postpartum care, and in other times of need.

ACUPUNCTURE

Acupuncture is one of the earliest forms of medicine, dating to around 100 BCE and referenced in the text *The Yellow Emperor's Classic of Internal Medicine.* This system of medicine diagnoses and treats the body based on elements found in nature that are the same as those found in the human body. By taking a detailed history of the patient and performing tongue diagnosis and pulse diagnosis, acupuncturists can identify areas of the body that are out of balance. They then create a treatment plan that calls for specific needle placements within the body to support the healthy flow of energy, referred to as Qi or Chi. When the elements and temperaments are in balance, Qi flows freely and supports optimal health through a system similar to the circulatory system. It's made of small channels called *nadis,* which make up the system that integrates incoming Qi into the physical body. When there is stagnation in the movement of Qi, disease can manifest, leading to pain, reduced organ function, chronic infections, buildup of toxins, mood changes, and chronic fatigue.

Acupuncturists study for years to memorize the meridian system, which took centuries to map. Meridians are pathways that run throughout the body, and each of the meridians is related to certain organ systems. Meridians are condensed lines of force running through the body from a collection of nadis. Think of this in terms of the human circulatory system, where the capillaries are the nadis and the meridians are the larger vessels the capillaries feed into.

The most common question patients ask about acupuncture is if the needles are big and if they hurt. I have experienced minor discomfort during acupuncture, but not because of the needles' size—they are about the width of a human hair—but because the imbalance in my system was responding to the treatment. The acupuncture needle redirects stagnant energy so it flows more freely to the organ system, thus improving the physical health of the organ as well as any mental-emotional stagnation associated with the imbalance. In acupuncture a physical needle is directed into the skin, but the energy it impacts has implications for the mind, body, and soul.

For those with tick-borne disease, acupuncture can enhance the healing process by reducing pain due to inflammation, improving detoxification, healing injuries, stabilizing sleep patterns, and creating space for self-care. Most insurance companies include coverage for acupuncture, and it is becoming more integrated into the conventional medical model each day.

CUPPING

Another modality associated with traditional Chinese medicine is cupping, a treatment in which small cauldron-like glass or soft plastic bulbs are placed on the skin, creating suction. This therapy is used to improve microcirculation of the capillaries, decrease toxins, and reduce tension and pain in the muscles.

The most popular method is dry cupping: A therapist puts a small amount of methylated ethers or another flammable substance into a glass cup and ignites it; when the flame goes out, he puts the cup upside down on the skin, creating a vacuum inside the cup. Alternatively, plastic cups with a suction device attached may be used to create a vacuum. Cups can be left in one place or dragged over oiled tissue to loosen tension for a short period of time. Depending on the level of suction, there can be some discomfort, but good communication with your practitioner will allow him to apply an ideal force. Cupping is another way of mobilizing stagnant blood flow and Qi energy flow in the body to improve health. It's enhanced when partnered with massage therapy.

Cupping gained sudden attention when, with the world watching, Michael Phelps appeared on the pool deck at the Olympics with red rings on his body that looked like bruises. This is a common outcome with cupping. The dark lesion is related to the level of stagnation in the tissue where the cups were applied. These marks are commonly not painful, as bruises are, but can look ominous for a few days after treatment.

MOXIBUSTION

Moxibustion is the application of burning dried moxa (*Artemisia vulgaris*) on or near the skin—smoke and heat emanate from the moxa much like from an incense stick. Moxa is typically hovered above acupuncture meridian points to stimulate the area and move stagnating energy. Its therapeutic benefit is related to aromatherapy from the smoke, heat, and location of the application. Research has validated the use of moxabustion to relieve irritable bowel syndrome, hypertension, and pain-related issues, and to reduce symptoms associated with cancer treatment, reduce swelling, and stimulate the immune system.[4] It is equally effective in treating pain and digestive issues and providing the immune support required in patients suffering from tick-borne infection.

FLOTATION THERAPY

Commonly referred to as flotation restricted environmental stimulation technique (REST) or sensory deprivation therapy, this technique has been around since the 1950s. The process involves lying face up in a quiet, darkened pod filled with highly concentrated magnesium sulfate–saturated water. This solution has a higher salt concentration than the Dead Sea, in which humans are completely buoyant. One can relax each and every muscle in a solitary, weightless state. Earplugs further reduce the intake of sensory information, contributing to the sense of calm.

The sensory deprivation tank was initially developed by medical doctor and neuropsychiatrist John Lilly in 1954. His studies focused on generating altered states of consciousness when sight, sound, and touch were dramatically diminished. This therapy has historically been more popular in Europe, but it is popping up in the United States in alternative health clinics as a method of relaxation, chronic disease management, and self-care.

Flotation REST therapy has been researched for several decades, mostly looking at its application for treating trauma, managing pain, enhancing sleep quality, and improving attention and cognition. It's been helpful in reducing pain from headaches, fibromyalgia, and premenstrual syndrome.

Researchers hypothesize that the pain-reducing effects arise from the body's naturally occurring endorphins, endocannabinoid system, and opioid system, and from a reduction in stress hormones.[5] Studies also show that the treatment brings people into a sleep state in which their brain wave function is equal to Sleep Stage 1, equivalent to a cat nap.[6] In this sleep stage, alpha and theta waves start to rise and changes in eye movement occur. Alpha waves are associated with a relaxed and contemplative state of mind, while theta waves bring you closer to the dreaming state, though you are still conscious. (Delta waves are the ones associated with deep sleep.)

The theta state is one of deep relaxation, and it can enhance creativity and the positive qualities of the right brain to put us more in tune with emotions, the whole picture, and intuition, as well as compassionate thinking for self and others. This enhanced right-brain activity creates more balance with the left-brain analytical mind, which excels at linear thinking, and is outcome driven and attached to time. Both hemispheres serve a purpose, and when the two are well synchronized, we have greater potential for improved mental health, increased neuroplasticity, and better overall mental processing. This translates into better health of the body, with balanced endocrine function and enhanced immunity.

Massage Therapy and Musculoskeletal Manipulation

Many people think of massage therapy as an indulgence, and some are afraid to get their bones adjusted. I can tell you that therapeutic touch can make an enormous difference in your ability to heal, as it can aid in detoxifying, improve blood flow to the brain, reduce stress, and improve the efficacy of medications.

One of the core symptoms in patients with tick-borne infections is pain. This usually manifests as muscle pain or nerve pain, with reduced flexibility. Some form of therapeutic touch is important to recovery, as it improves blood circulation in the tissues. In fact, the connective tissues in your body, called

Some form of therapeutic touch is important to recovery, as it improves blood circulation in the tissues.

fascia, cover the muscles throughout your body and work as a whole system. They communicate through Bonghan ducts, which transmit information in a circulatory system independent of the blood or lymphatic circulatory systems.[7] These channels send signals to enhance tissue repair and development based on the needs of the body, and they have an impact on connective tissue, muscles, bone, and neurological tissue. Stagnation in the tissues creates the perfect ground for infection and toxins, which can certainly disrupt proper communication.

Massage helps improve the flow of communication, since this circulatory system is promoted by movement of the tissues.

When a muscle holds tension due to a hypervigilant nervous system, this tension restricts blood, creating an area of hypoxia (low-oxygen environment). In this state of low oxygen, inflammation triggers muscles and nerves, causing pain. This type of pain is referred to as *myofascial pain syndrome* and typically manifests with a number of trigger points. These trigger points can refer pain to outlying areas, making it difficult to know where the origin of the pain is. As the tension stays in the muscle, the muscle will pull the bones out of alignment, and this misalignment creates even more muscle pain. Compensation in the body can lead to imbalances in the right and left sides, as well as problems with posture. Carrying pain in this way often leads to reduced activity levels, which only feeds the cycle. Thus, bringing bones back into alignment with a visit to a chiropractor, osteopathic physician, or naturopathic doctor can be most beneficial.

The marriage of these two modalities is critical: If the underlying tension in the muscle is not addressed with massage and you just receive adjustments, muscle tension will keep pulling the bones out of place. However, if you only treat with massage and an area continues to be a problem despite adequate attention, you may require a realignment to allow the tension to release in the muscle. At the core of all this is mitigating stress with mindfulness and moderation in lifestyle choices, which can help prevent tension from accruing in the first place.

Before moving on, let's address the possibility of experiencing a Herxheimer reaction with both these hands-on treatments. The likelihood of this response is because of the increase in blood flow, which liberates toxins and disturbs pockets of tissue where spirochetes are making their home. As these are released into the system, a flare or even a fever may follow. In my early twenties, before I contracted Lyme disease, I went for my first deep tissue massage. At the time, I lived in Los Angeles, where there were many places to receive alternative healing therapies. A couple of hours after the massage was over, I felt nauseated, with flulike symptoms, and had to stay home the next day to recover. I saw this negatively then and never wanted to get a massage again. However, I later learned this was normal and beneficial, and I was happy those toxins I had been walking around with were gone.

Massage and bone adjustments vary in intensity based on the practitioner's training. Traditional massage sessions, sought for relaxation, are at one end of the spectrum while at the other end are more intense forms, such as Rolfing. Rolfing involves the massage therapist applying deep, slow-moving pressure to break up the fascia sheaths around the muscles, as these become adhered and calcified over time. Rolfing can bring about profound changes in posture, release toxins, and release emotional memory held in the muscle. Emotional muscle memory can manifest with any therapeutic touch, but it seems to be released especially with Rolfing or other techniques that break up fascia. This can come up as spontaneous release of emotion and flashes of memories. I won't sugarcoat it; it's physically uncomfortable. But deep tissue work can be well worth it when you feel ready; it can be beneficial in creating proper alignment in the body, which decreases pain and improves internal organ function.

Craniosacral Work

Neurological impairments involving cognition, abnormal body movements, visual changes, ringing in the ears, pressure in the head, and vertigo are all common symptoms of Lyme disease that make daily life difficult for the average patient. These symptoms can be due to impaired flow of cerebrospinal fluid, which runs throughout the brain spaces and the spinal column in a system considered a third circulatory system (the first two are those carrying blood and lymphatic fluid).

The craniosacral system is devoted to cleansing, protecting, and nourishing the organs of the central nervous system. This includes the brain, the covering over the brain (the meninges), the spinal column, and the glial cells. When the flow of cerebrospinal fluid is healthy, it moves through the deeper aspects of the brain via a system of channels, washing over the surface of the brain and down the column of the spinal cord. This fluid does not have the same velocity as blood moving through the circulatory system but is affected by reverberations from the heartbeat. With stress, infection, inflammation, or head injury (major or minor), the flow of cerebrospinal fluid can be disrupted.

Craniosacral work uses subtle touch and traction to feel areas of tension associated with the fascia of the skull and spinal cord. The level of touch is

Sauna Therapy

HEAT THERAPIES ARE IDEAL FOR THOSE WHO CAN TOLERATE THEM. I know many Lyme disease patients have a hard time in the heat and flat out don't like it. Sauna therapy, or therapeutic sweating, has been used in numerous cultures for thousands of years for its health benefits, and it has ceremonial uses and a social aspect as well. The sauna design most commonly seen today, with the wooden walls and heated stone, has its origins in Finland. If you are purchasing a sauna for your home, please make sure the wood is free of the toxins found in treated wood, which would inevitably off-gas in the box and create more toxins in your body.

Traditional saunas, heated with stones, raise the core body temperature to create a feverlike response in the body, which clears toxins and enhances the immune system's ability to clear infections. The idea is to have a dry environment so heat can be maximally effective, since water on the skin has a cooling effect. A steam room does not provide the same benefits and is actually a breeding ground for pathogens. Ideally, the inside temperature is 110°F–160°F (43°C–71°C)—most are around 120°F (49°C). If you have never tried a sauna before, your initial sitting should be approximately five minutes. Bring plenty of water to drink while in the sauna and continue to drink afterward to rehydrate. Toxins will be emitted from your skin, and you will experience upregulating in the enzyme pathway, triggered by heat.

A related therapy developed in Japan, called *Waon therapy*, uses a dry sauna set at about 130°F (54°C) for ten to fifteen minutes followed by a thirty-minute body wrap in heated blankets to maintain the internal body temperature for the hyperthermic effects.[8] This process has been seen to improve chronic fatigue, decrease pain associated with fibromyalgia, improve depressed moods, and improve hypertension.[9] Waon therapy is similar to hot fomentation, a hydrotherapy treatment that also involves wrapping a patient with layers of sheets, wool blankets, and hot packs to increase the core body temperature and clear infections.

Infrared saunas, which utilize an infrared bulb to create heat, are now available in the form of a cabinet you sit in, a bodysuit you zip up, or lamps that project localized heat to activate a specific area of the body. Three different forms of light are emitted in the infrared spectrum—these are near infrared, middle infrared, and far infrared. Far infrared, the type used for therapeutic value, has the ability to penetrate 0.8–1.2 inches (2–3 cm) into tissue without causing burns or negative side effects. While the mechanism is not fully understood, studies have shown improved circulation, reduced pain, enhanced energy levels, and improved insulin metabolism.[10]

very gentle compared with the typical pressure used in massage therapy. Practitioners are trained to apply pressure to specific locations until they become aware of the fascia releasing, thus allowing unimpeded flow of cerebrospinal fluid. This can also lead to subtle changes in the bones of the head. The sutures of the brain, long thought to solidify after early childhood, still make very slight movements to adjust for pressure within the head while maintaining strength to protect the delicate brain.

Restriction in the flow of cerebrospinal fluid can cause impaired functioning of motor neurons, sensory neurons, and the sympathetic and parasympathetic nervous systems. Impaired flow has a dramatic impact on the glial cells, which make up a majority of the brain mass and have important functions in maintaining homeostasis in the brain. They form the protective myelin sheaths around nerves, help hold nerves in place, detect imbalances in the brain, attack invading microbes, oxygenate neurons, play an important role in our ability to breathe properly, and keep order in the brain.

If you are experiencing stress to the nervous system, you might find it helpful to seek out a practitioner trained in craniosacral work. This will typically be a massage therapist, chiropractor, osteopath, or another practitioner trained in administering physical medicine modalities. Treatment in this modality could decrease Herxing symptoms and help with recovery. Research has already documented its benefits to those who have suffered concussion or who have persistent headaches, traumatic brain injury, or debilitating back pain.

In Summary

Chronic illnesses such as Lyme disease mean that the body is a very uncomfortable place to be. And if the body is uncomfortable, it can be hard to see the possibility of recovery. You can get stuck in pain cycles, physically, mentally, and emotionally. Engaging in some form of self-care, whatever is physically possible, can change your outlook dramatically by enhancing neurotransmitters, improving the flexibility of your body by enhancing circulation, and creating a deeper mind-body connection.

Physical medicine is about regrowing the body you desire for the future. Start simple and keep showing up for yourself daily with some form of activity, no matter how minimal it may seem. Engaging in self-care to strengthen, lengthen, and relax your body is an act of intention designed to heal. Repeating the activity you choose with patience will signal your body to make positive changes.

3

WHEN LYME PERSISTS: IT'S TIME TO DIG DEEP

CHAPTER 10

THE NEW NORMAL: LIVING WITH CHRONIC LYME DISEASE

Y ou finally have a diagnosis that explains your multitude of symptoms. You have an answer. Tears flow, and with them comes relief. But relief is followed by trepidation about what's to come. What will the future look like? You waited so long for the answer—and questions arise about why it was so hard to find. Why didn't other doctors address your symptoms and concerns? Why were you forced to go from one doctor and treatment to another, looking for relief? These are not easy questions to answer, but it is helpful to acknowledge that, as I've mentioned before, there is a distinct pushback in parts of the medical community regarding a diagnosis of chronic Lyme disease.

Now that Lyme disease and other tick-borne infections are part of your life, you may experience Lyme disease culture shock. Chronic Lyme disease has its own nuances of terminology, process of recovery, socioeconomic impact, and unique presentations based on age and gender. In addition, a diagnosis of Lyme disease brings its own set of emotions that rise up and lead to certain changes within the individual and in family dynamics. Many variables affect the duration of recovery, the treatment and circumstances it takes to recover, and the ways in which a patient's life will change for a period of time.

Providing encouragement for my patients is where I spend a lot of time during office visits, but it is so necessary for patient recovery. My office is a safe space where patients do not need to explain themselves or defend their diagnosis. Knowing this, patients often start to cry. The stress can be overwhelming after they have felt sick for so long and have dealt with confusion, doubts, and a fear that they will never get their quality of life back, coupled with the strain of maintaining an appearance of regular life. Patients' worries are often compounded by the stress on their caretakers, who are frequently overlooked but may work themselves to the bone to help their loved ones. The lives of caretakers can change dramatically, too, particularly if income levels in the house drop because not only the patient but also the caretaker is unable to work due to the needs of the patient.

So many variables make having chronic Lyme disease more difficult than it needs to be, and we have discussed many of them throughout this book. One of the most common conversations I have with patients concerns the reasons their primary care doctors did not acknowledge their Lyme disease. Polarized opinions of doctors regarding chronic Lyme disease confuse patients, who lose touch with their intuition because for so long they have seen specialists, emergency room doctors, and primary care providers who tell them nothing is wrong except anxiety.

After a formal diagnosis of chronic Lyme disease, patients need time to deprogram; though they'd experienced ongoing symptoms, they had convinced themselves that everything was in their head, based on what others told them. Now they have developed trauma, anxiety, and possibly even psychosis because of the labels applied to them. It was just easier to accept mental imbalance as their reality.

The task of helping patients overcome medical trauma can also make being a Lyme-literate doctor difficult, as we must manage conflicting information in the media about Lyme disease. We also tend to take the brunt of the emotions from patients as they process feelings of confusion and betrayal. I spend a lot of time addressing new therapies patients read about in blogs, consoling those who have had confrontations with doctors, and coaching patients through Herxheimer reactions made worse by stress. All of this causes patients to second-guess their treatment plan, which leads to doctor-hopping as they explore the wide variety of treatments with differing philosophies, price points, and promises of cure.

Discussing the plight of those who suffer from chronic Lyme disease and other tick-borne infections is a service to those who are not being heard. I want to address here the trauma aligned with the label chronic Lyme disease and emphasize the way it integrates with the trauma a person carried before diagnosis. While not everyone who has Lyme disease has trauma, many do.

Just enduring the medical difficulties we've discussed, living with symptoms and prolonged debilitation, and trying to find a treating doctor can be traumatic. My contribution with this book is to acknowledge patients' experiences and open a dialogue to advance understanding of this complex disease.

I want to emphasize that I am not a licensed counselor or therapist. My undergraduate degree is in psychology, and before attending medical school, I worked for several years in social work with at-risk populations—including those who were homeless, escaping violent homes, or suicidal—and I advocated on behalf of those in crisis after a rape. I have spent several years in medical practice, providing counsel and referral for patients going through personal difficulties and have had many discussions regarding their personal safety and intent to harm themselves. I have also worked in conjunction with counselors in a team approach, providing a safe space for patients to talk about trauma and discussing coping mechanisms they can integrate into their daily lives. Working with those who have tick-borne diseases involves counseling patients daily. However, it's important to have licensed mental health professional on board who can support patients throughout their treatment.

Trauma and Tick-Borne Disease

Trauma is derived from a Greek word meaning "a wound," and in psychological terms, it means "witnessing or experiencing a horrifying or shocking event and feeling intense fear or helplessness afterward." The latest edition of the *Diagnostic and Statistical Manual of Mental Disorders* (DSM-5) features the most expansive criteria for post-traumatic stress disorder (PTSD); until this edition, a diagnosis of PTSD had been highly controversial, even though most patients who seek counseling have past trauma as defined by the manual. We have all had trauma at one time or another, and it does not have to be extreme to qualify because a trauma is subjective. Severity and duration, however, can determine the intervention required.

While the wounds created by trauma can be physical, the physical wounds heal; mental-emotional wounds can remain for a lifetime if they are not resolved. How well trauma is resolved depends on the support the person receives after the event(s) and on the person's resilience, which makes the path highly individualized. Through the processes of dissociation (disconnecting from thoughts, feelings, or memories), repression, and fragmentation, our traumatic events can be stored in the shadows of the mind—these are part of

Thankfully, due to neuro-plasticity... we can rewire our responses and heal from trauma.

humans' natural survival mechanisms. These mechanisms represent an important process of coping rather than a weakness or a failure. However, when these coping mechanisms outlive their usefulness (helping us survive) and become a source of more suffering, the condition is diagnosed as PTSD.

Dissociation is related to fragmentation, in which thoughts and actions are split. When someone witnesses something shocking, his mind tries to minimize suffering and ensure survival by repressing the event (excluding the thoughts from the conscious mind), losing memories of the situation, and/or creating altered versions of the story. A traumatized person may also feel numb or detached from his body. As the trauma continues, the memories or parts of the psyche can fragment, splitting off into pieces, because the reality being presented does not make sense or is intolerable. These pieces are banished to the unconscious mind but can reemerge later.

In some circumstances, detachment or dissociation can be a healthy process, as this helps us maintain proper boundaries in our relationships and in our interactions with the world. For instance, you could feel an emotional punch to the gut after seeing a news story. You can either stay with those feelings or detach from them. You can't fix all the suffering in the world. In this situation, you might dissociate from the news story and instead do your best to create positive change around you.

Fragmentation is the breaking down of memories so they are not accessible. This is most common after prolonged childhood trauma, where a person forms a new personality out of a necessity for survival. Fragmentation can thus lead a person to be detached, numb, emotionally unstable, perfection driven, codependent, anxious, outgoing, or gregarious. There also may be no perceptible sign of a person's wounds. The way people cope with trauma is extremely diverse and is based on individual circumstances and particular psychological makeup. Some may rise above the trauma into a lighter state of being, while others sink deeper into darkness. Often, the same person will be involved in an ongoing process of visiting the extremes of both worlds.

A child's brain is like a sponge, and primitive survival mechanisms can bury traumas deep in the brain if the child does not have the language or context to process the event fully. Children deal with unloving acts, pain, and shocking events by trying to make sense of them, often by creating a belief that the event was their fault, feeling deep shame, or hiding their resentment of others. Thankfully, due to neuroplasticity (our brains' ability to change), we can rewire our responses and heal from trauma. This is usually done with the help of others in the medical, psychological, and/or spiritual field who can help us access memories while ensuring that we remain stable.

I gather a trauma history for almost every new patient. Initially, the patient may not feel comfortable sharing these experiences. When I ask patients if they have experienced any traumatic moments, many will first say no but will then launch into deeply troubling experiences. They may claim that these experiences are resolved or that they did not consider the situations traumatic when compared with things that have happened to others. They tell their stories with little to no emotion, or even make light of them—including stories of abuse, near-death situations, sexual trauma, medical trauma, neglect, military trauma, extreme violence, loss of loved ones, homelessness, drug addiction, incest, and more.

Many patients see little or no correlation between their current situation and past trauma. Discussing the role of trauma in chronic Lyme disease is tricky because of the risk that the patient will lose trust in me if they feel I am saying the disease is largely a mental-emotional problem. Also, it is important to let the patient take back his power in the situation; it is my role to provide an opening for discussion but not to force or coax information about past trauma from them.

POST-TRAUMATIC STRESS DISORDER AND CHRONIC LYME DISEASE

PTSD commonly affects the Lyme disease treatment process, as old wounds are reopened and are compounded by increased inflammation in the brain due to the microbial infection. It can be very difficult for patients to wade through painful emotions while recovering from an infection. Many report a fear of being watched, recurrent nightmares, fear of the outside environment, and, of course, fear of bugs. In several cases, patients have developed agoraphobia after being isolated for a long period of time and spending so much time at home. They can have unpredictable physical spells such as seizures, problems with speech, debilitating hypersensitivity to light or sounds, or fainting spells.

Patients also experience flashbacks, emotional overreactions to small stressors, bursts of anger, violence, obsessive thoughts, self-medicating, thoughts of harm, and self-abuse. These intense reactions are then followed by sorrow, shame, and embarrassment. They are shocked by their own behavior or feelings because these reactions are contrary to their normal behavior; they feel as if someone else took over. Extreme reactions are not necessarily trauma driven, but reactions from neuroinflammation can create future traumas that require care if they are not addressed appropriately at the time of the incident. This is especially difficult with younger children, who can't fully understand why they are feeling or acting this way. PTSD affects relationships within families, with friends and coworkers, and especially with partners.

There are many similarities between those with PTSD and those with chronic Lyme disease. Both tend to experience loss of friendships, social networks, and jobs as well as higher divorce rates. They often have reduced social support because of the ongoing nature of the illness; friends and acquaintances fall away because of their own difficulties in holding space with someone who is chronically ill. It's hard for relationships to hold steady when one person changes dramatically. The person who is ill may be unable to participate in the activities that gave the relationship its connection.

Being chronically ill and trapped in a sick body causes old fears to reemerge in many patients. Denial of the illness by a medical doctor and/or Herxheimer reactions lead the patient to feel victimized or abused all over again. Patients with chronic Lyme disease and other tick-borne diseases who have unresolved trauma are my most debilitated population, taking years to recover, with more intense neurological presentations that limit their physical, mental, and emotional function. They tend to be more sensitive to medications, have frequent relapses, are unable to emotionally tolerate Herxheimer reactions, and often abandon treatment because of a heightened fight-or-flight response.

Those suffering from both PTSD and chronic Lyme disease may feel that they can't trust their own bodies. The risk of being seen in public in a vulnerable state limits these patients' outings, further isolating them. This can lead to profound loneliness and a sense of being shut in by their failing body. People who loved the outdoors may become petrified to go outside for any length of time, for fear of getting a tick bite. Even a short trip to the mailbox can cause panic. People who were outdoor enthusiasts no longer do what they love out of fear of being bitten again.

SUICIDE RISK

One of my main motivations for writing this book is the harsh reality that chronic Lyme disease patients struggling with the illness may begin to think of suicide. In an article titled "Suicide and Lyme and Associated Diseases," Robert Bransfield, M.D., reports a high level of suicidal ideation in Lyme disease patients. He correlates suicide attempts with neurocognitive changes in the brain, due to increased neuroinflammation, that cause thoughts of self-harm. In addition, negative attitudes toward chronic Lyme disease sufferers cause patients to feel alienated.[1] The fact is, most people who die from Lyme disease and associated coinfections die by their own hand. It's a heavy burden to carry the disease and defend it at the same time. But this does not have to be the reality; much suffering could be eliminated if patients, families, the medical community, and government approached patients with greater compassion and inclusivity.

Suicidal ideation is nondiscriminatory—it affects those of all ages and genders. I have seen children diagnosed with Lyme disease and pediatric autoimmune neuropsychiatric disorders associated with streptococcal infections (PANDAS) who show cutting behaviors, have thoughts of suicide, or exhibit other forms of self-harm, necessitating psychiatric care. Children and adults with no apparent history before contracting tick-borne disease become suicide risks. While a great deal of detail about PANDAS is beyond the scope of this book, it's important to screen children who may be affected for strepto-coccal antibodies, along with testing for tick-borne disease, especially if a patient exhibits psychiatric symptoms after the onset of fever, sore throat, confirmed strep infection, or flulike symptoms.

The stigma surrounding chronic Lyme disease creates an atmosphere in which patients feel the need to hide symptoms, which enhances stress and shame. Among the lowest emotional states, shame involves humiliation and isolation and can bring one eventually to thoughts of self-harm just to end the suffering. This is mostly due to prolonged pain, mental and emotional imbal-ance, and isolation; but these symptoms could largely be avoided if we ended the social rejection of those who have chronic Lyme disease and funded education for the general public to foster greater compassion and awareness.

Resisting Counseling When It's Needed Most

At the core of trauma as it interacts with chronic Lyme is fear and the hyper-vigilance that comes from feeling that we live in an unsafe world. If the body feels unsafe, it will respond with an impulse to escape or to freeze, whether the threat is real or imagined. For many, the train tracks for these behaviors were laid long before Lyme disease came along, and the process of treatment and recovery acted as an emotional trigger that brought those feelings to the surface. If this happens, it is important to have proper psychological and social support in place. Leaping into trauma work at a vulnerable time is not always something a patient is ready to do, and that is okay. Everything has its unique timing. My job as a doctor is to have the dialogue, open the door to the possibil-ities, and then help the patient find the most appropriate treatment option.

While we may associate the ability to keep moving on with strength, all we do when we do not treat trauma is compartmentalize the pain to be experi-enced in the future. This affects our daily life, certainly, but unresolved PTSD can also increase anxiety, depression, and mood imbalance in offspring even one or two generations later, referred to as *transgenerational trauma* (I will discuss this more later in the chapter).[2]

Many patients resist the idea of seeing a counselor until they are brought to a point of surrender; they must nearly break down before they can see the connections between their current health and the old wounds that haunt them. Avoidance of counseling can also be due to a person's general opinions about its efficacy; her gender, age, or fear of being vulnerable; associated costs; and concern about the time it will take. The biggest concern a patient may have is that she will see a therapist who does not believe she has Lyme disease. This, again, comes from the medical trauma of being humiliated or disbelieved by other practitioners.

I let people know it's not important that a counselor understand Lyme disease, although that is helpful. What is critical is that the counselor is trained in trauma work and family counseling and that he or she is compassionate. Counseling offers an opportunity to process emotions and gain skills needed to cope with a difficult life situation.

Every person's timing is different with regard to their call to do trauma work. A health crisis can be a turning point that presents an amazing opportunity to change. I have seen profound changes in people who have rigid defense mechanisms, and who refuse to see their illness as anything but a purely physical problem. Eventually, though, they soften and begin to open themselves to receiving help. The ability to ask for help, receive help, and be okay with being vulnerable are some of the major emotional blocks that Lyme disease patients experience. When they do allow themselves to receive help, they heal much more efficiently. This does not mean recovery is easy, but they experience breakthroughs so strong that, even if the body is not fully recovered, they can improve self-care and feel greater joy and peace. It's amazing to watch a person find her grace.

Your Trauma Is Not Yours Alone

Trauma has many layers and different origins: There is individual trauma, transgenerational trauma, and collective trauma. These are defined separately but can overlap throughout life. The way we are affected by one trauma affects how we handle others. Individual trauma is what we experience in this lifetime based on what happens to us directly. Living in the world means we are going to see, hear, and feel difficult things. These experiences shape our reality—our view of our surroundings and the people we meet. However, this view was set in motion by our families and our culture.

Grassroots Efforts to Create Community Support

IN MY AREA OF SOUTHERN NEW HAMPSHIRE, I have watched grassroots support groups create networks that help Lyme disease patients find others who understand their journey and exchange names of doctors who will treat them. These networks are like local chronic Lyme disease phone trees. Typically, if someone is even minimally vocal about having recovered from Lyme disease, they get flooded with emails, phone calls, and inquiries. They become an information, referral, and support network as well as a crisis line. Many of my patients formed relationships in my waiting room and while receiving intravenous therapy in my IV suite. They banded together to create a support group so they could balance the workload of all the community support they were already doing from their own homes. They rotate meetings at different homes a few times each month.

TRANSGENERATIONAL TRAUMA

We have focused on individual trauma throughout much of this chapter, but most of us come from families with many generations of trauma. Transgenerational traumas are those that have been passed down from generation to generation. These might include, for example, your family migrating to a different continent and barely scraping by. Such an experience can dramatically affect a whole family and change the way individuals will parent. They may pass their fear of scarcity down to future generations. This fear can move through several generations, until no one really knows why they have certain tendencies; they just report that being depressed, angry, or anxious runs in the family. Experience of scarcity can manifest as worry over not having enough, fear of failure, overindulgence, hoarding, or fear of spending money, which limits enjoyment. This is just one example of a core transgenerational trauma centered around survival and primitive needs.

Family Constellation Work, developed by Bert Hellinger in the 1990s, is a method of healing unhealthy family patterns. This work is done in a group therapy setting; the group does not need to be related or even know one another. As the therapy session opens, the group will start to gain insight into the origins of the conflict that affects a seeker (a person looking for help) from the perspective of their ancestors, as data start to emerge through the group. The group is accessing the unconscious information field of the seeker's family in order to identify the origins of unhealthy patterns that have moved through generations. Groups are facilitated by trained counselors who help maintain emotional safety throughout the process. For more information on healing transgenerational trauma, consult Mark Wolynn's *It Didn't Start with You: How Inherited Family Trauma Shapes Who We Are and How to End the Cycle*.

Recently, a patient of mine attended a group session in Family Constellation Work. She reported that those who have chronic Lyme disease also have conflict rooted in being without a clan. I had to sit with that for a while because at first the connection was difficult to make. Being without a clan relates to loss of family identity, feelings of aloneness, lack of support and group protection, and feelings of being essentially cut off. Humans used to be heavily associated with their group identity—with their tribe, clan, and the land. I find it interesting that the *Borrelia* spirochete moves from mammal to tick back to mammal. It is constantly being moved from one extreme environment to the next. It is drawn in by the tick, harbored, then pushed back out again to start anew. I feel there is a connection between the energy of the microbe and our own inner conflict of being without the support we may need within our family unit. I'll talk about the relationship of microbes and inner conflict more in the final chapter of the book.

Again, it's important to remember, when speaking from a transgenerational perspective, that your family may have a loving and supportive structure, but if we were to look several generations back, there may be unconscious inner conflict that affects your health today.

Researchers are using animal models such as mice to watch the changes in successive generations, observing both negative and positive outcomes from stressors in their ancestors. They are also studying the impact of trauma on gametes (sperm/egg) and genetic alterations that happen in utero. The point of this research is to understand observable biological changes rather than relying solely on a psychological perspective. We also need to know if successive generations can reverse these pathways and how they heal them over time. Can traumas in fact help later generations develop adaptability to stress?

Most research in trauma and epigenetics is done by creating trauma in mice and then watching successive generations respond to the trauma. Researchers track genetic markers associated with PTSD and mental illness, such as the FKBP5 gene, and they watch modification through methylation. Replicating this type of study in humans would not be ethical, of course, but longitudinal studies have followed those who have survived horrific trauma, such as the Holocaust, and looked at the genetic changes in their offspring. Those who survived the Holocaust had an upregulation of genes triggered by PTSD as well as those that affect stress hormone release and mood disorders, as would be expected. Then researchers found that this same gene was altered in the survivors' offspring but in a dramatically different way.[3] Researchers are continuing to work in this area to understand how the genetic makeup of offspring are affected by changes to the parents' genes.

COLLECTIVE TRAUMA

Collective trauma is the wave of energy that moves through a large group of people and engenders a collective fear based on a trial experienced by the group. This creates a change in culture that can take generations to heal because of the large scale of the event and the depth of the fear or pain. War, genocide, and environmental calamity are all examples of events that can lead to collective trauma. In the information age, we have greater awareness than ever before of the suffering in the world, and many of us are affected by the ills of other cultures that we would not have known about in previous decades or centuries.

When embarking on trauma work, you may have emotions rise up in your awareness that are not relevant to your current life but which may have been part of a pattern held in your cellular structure over generations. Fear of scarcity, a feeling of not having a homeland, shame, shock, grief, addictions, attachments, and a feeling of not living up to expectations are just a few of the emotions we may experience. We can heal with conscious effort, but we need to understand that it's normal to have these feelings emerge. It's also helpful to work with a counselor or other practitioner who can guide you through the healing process as gracefully as possible.

Your Brain Is Plastic

Fortunately, we humans are highly adaptable, not only as a species but on an individual level as well. Neuroplasticity is the ability of our nerve synapses to regrow based on learned behavior. For many years, scientists believed that the brain could not be changed, that it operates in a fixed way. The acceptance of neuroplasticity—the ability of the nervous system to reorganize itself in response to injury, illness, sensory data, developmental changes, or damage—represents a big shift in this long-held belief. Nerves form new synapses and branches to relay sensory information; these branches are also pruned back by microglia to maintain efficiency when they are no longer of use because positive changes have occurred or due to injury.

Your brain's plasticity is the reason that it is important, if you want to regain or enhance function, to continually expose your body and/or mind to the desired experience; this sends a message to the system that these neuronal branches are necessary. For example, to regain strength or endurance, don't wait until you feel strong enough to do a task. Start the process, no matter how minimal, to create the body strength you desire.

> **To regain strength or endurance,** don't wait until you feel strong enough to do a task. Start the process, no matter how minimal, to create the body strength you desire.

The same is true for developing better memory. You need to engage in the activity to regrow new neurons. This can be retraining your brain with programs such as those available through Lumosity (www.lumosity.com), using the opposing hand for basic tasks (if you are right dominant, then use your left hand to brush your teeth), learning new skills, reading, and writing. Set aside judgment of the outcome; your result is not about being graded but about the doing.

In his book *The Biology of Belief*, Bruce Lipton, Ph.D., discusses in depth the amazing ability of the body to heal and rewire itself based on new stimuli. Many other practitioners and scientists have also understood this, as have traditional healers throughout the ages. As we heal our wounds, we have limitless potential for positive changes and for growth of new neurons better aligned with healthy thinking, feeling, and mind-body connection. To learn more about neuroplasticity, read *The Brain That Changes Itself*, by Norman Doidge, M.D.

Epigenetics: Finding Our On-Off Switch

The initial theory of genetics, now disregarded, is referred to as *preformation*. Under this theory, we are born with everything we will need carried in the embryo, and these traits gradually reveal themselves over a lifetime, with no variability.

Epigenesis is now the more accepted viewpoint. *Epigenetics*, a term first introduced in 1942 by embryologist and developmental biologist Conrad Waddington, is the ability of our environment to influence our bodies as we move through our lives.[4] Our genetic code is the blueprint for cellular growth, development, and regeneration as well as eventual degeneration. Our DNA sequence can't be altered, but it can adapt during our lifetime.

This "study above our genes"—*epi* means "on" or "above"—involves research into the proteins responsible for turning genes on or off based on our diet, sleep quality, lifestyle choices, stressors, traumas, and beliefs. These are all areas over which we have control. DNA is like a tightly wound circuit board that can be activated or deactivated based on messages received from the external environment. Certain mechanisms—two of the most researched are methyl groups (an alkyl derived from methane) and histones (proteins found in chromatin)—can turn genes on and off; they can silence a gene, subtly enhance it, or activate it, depending on the needs of the body as well as response to stressors.

Here, we will quickly revisit microglial cells (immune cells of the brain) because a lot of research is working to better understand their role in brain inflammation, studying pro-inflammatory pathways involved in Alzheimer's disease, drug addiction, strokes, multiple sclerosis, chronic Lyme disease, and several other conditions. It was once thought that microglial cells were largely inactive unless there was acute injury; however, research is showing that they are in constant movement, using methods of epigenetics such as methylation to implement action. The better we understand these mechanisms, the more effective our solutions to reduce the brain inflammation that causes debilitation.[5] Currently, little research is focusing on epigenetics and Lyme disease. Hopefully, this will change. The important takeaway here is that our immune response to Lyme disease spirochetes can be modified by our behaviors, diet, and management of stress. We have more control than we think.

Conversion Disorders and Psychosomatic Medicine

While we have great potential to adapt to our environment and heal ourselves from many illnesses, when our mind and body are out of balance, our ability to fight off disease and function optimally is curtailed. Many patients who come to my clinic have previously been given a diagnosis of psychosomatic manifestation of illness or conversion disorder. Psychosomatic illness is defined as a disease or disorder caused by, or made worse by, mental factors, including stress. A conversion disorder is a condition caused by mental factors but which takes on a neurological component such as fits of shaking, seizure-like activity, transitory blindness, and/or loss of sensation in the body. Symptoms listed above commonly occur in cases of tick-borne disease, as spirochetes can cause deterioration of nerves, depending on the host's immune system and stress.

I have treated multitudes of patients who have had a diagnosis of conversion disorder, which has been used to dismiss their symptoms and cause shame.

I have seen patients mentally and emotionally harmed when doctors tell them that they need to accept that they do not have Lyme disease and should instead seek a mental health practitioner or start taking a mood-stabilizing medication. This approach causes patients to feel humiliation and alienation, and it fosters negative thoughts. This experience causes further shame, aversion to seeking medical care, and increased suicidal ideation.

We need to understand more fully how the psyche holds on to negative beliefs, thoughts, and fears and how imprints from old traumas change the health of the physical body, making it more hospitable to illness. These are not new concepts, but they have gone in and out of favor over the past century as attitudes toward mental illness changed. The advent of psychiatric medications led to drugs becoming the primary answer to mental or emotional problems, when there is typically an underlying conflict that has not been addressed.

Psychosomatic medicine is really expanding in the medical field, blending several medical specialties, including psychology, psychophysiology, sociology, and psychoneuroimmunology (a focus on thoughts, beliefs, and emotions on the neurological and immunological systems).

Placebo and Nocebo Effects

When I was in medical school, I spent a lot of time in the library, as most medical students do. My favorite book was about five inches (13 cm) thick and was called *Spontaneous Remissions*. This book was filled with seemingly miraculous recoveries. I was intrigued by the countless case studies, written up by physicians and clinicians all over the world, of individuals who defied all odds by shrinking softball-size tumors with the belief they were being cured by trial medications, when in fact they were in the placebo group. (A placebo is a medication that has no therapeutic benefit other than the strong belief of the patient that it's beneficial.)

In the medical community, treatment response categorized as the *placebo effect* is often used to downplay the patient experience or the benefit of a medication. I most frequently hear about the placebo effect with regard to homeopathic medications, which are diluted substances that create changes in the system on the cellular level—or even the quantum level. While this certainly may seem to fit the criteria of a placebo, I have seen distinct and powerful healing outcomes with the use of homeopathic treatments. I personally think we just do not have technology that would allow us to fully witness how these medications work.

An Epidemic of Psychosomatic Disorders?

IF LYME DISEASE IS NOT THE PROBLEM, as many practitioners believe, we need to investigate the apparent epidemic of psychosomatic illness. Many patients are referred to a counselor, placed on medications for depression/anxiety, and told that all their problems are rooted in a psychiatric issue. Patients who choose not to accept this as their answer are still left with a worry in the back of their minds that they really are mentally ill, which only creates more inner turmoil.

Once a diagnosis of conversion disorder or psychosomatic illness is placed in a patient's chart, it follows him as he is referred to specialists such as neurologists, cardiologists, and so on. Accessibility to electronic records within hospital systems makes it even harder to escape the labels. Such a diagnosis has the power to change the perception of the next practitioner reviewing the case. Patients have reported, on many occasions, that doctors have either refused to see them after reviewing their charts, saying they couldn't help, or that it would be a waste of time for the patient to come in if the purpose is to discuss Lyme disease. While it may sound as though I am throwing the conventional medical community under the bus, I have great respect for the many medical doctors who are compassionate and open minded about chronic Lyme disease; however, the problems reported by hundreds of patients over the years who have visited multiple clinics and heard the same skeptical speech must be acknowledged before we can begin to change attitudes to better serve patients.

We also see an opposite of the placebo effect, called the *nocebo effect*. *Nocebo* actually means "I shall harm." This is a psychological manifestation rooted in negative experiences with medical intervention or medications, or in a general belief that something bad will happen. The nocebo effect has an important role in chronic Lyme disease treatment. After being diagnosed with Lyme disease, the first thing most patients do is search the Internet or talk to others about Lyme disease. As they hear or read other people's difficult stories, they form a belief that their own experience will be as challenging.

Our culture is highly ambivalent about medication: We are afraid to be without it, and at the same time we fear taking it. The television commercials drug companies produce to convince us we need their medications end in a rapid-fire list of horrifying side effects. Picking up medication at the pharmacy is likewise difficult, as we walk away with lengthy printouts detailing every possible calamity that could befall us if we take the drug.

When doctors support the patient's choice, even if they do not fully agree with the diagnosis, the patient experiences a better outcome.

Thus, the nocebo effect can be triggered by simply picking up the medication at the pharmacy or by Internet research. Many patients have an aversion to taking pills; they resent being tied to a medication regimen or are afraid because a medication caused an adverse event in the past. They project that negative feeling onto the new medication and expect it, too, to fail.

Anxiety and confusion in the medical community over chronic Lyme disease only amplifies these worries. Another significant cause of the nocebo effect is practitioners who disagree about whether chronic Lyme disease is real. When a patient has a negative interaction with a doctor such as his primary care provider about his Lyme treatment protocol, the doctor's attitude affects the patient's response to medication. It seeds doubts regarding the diagnosis and may eventually lead the patient to abandon treatment. When doctors support the patient's choice, even if they do not fully agree with the diagnosis, the patient experiences a better outcome.

The placebo and nocebo effects are where the power of intention meets science. Instead of thinking of these effects as an annoying extraneous factor in research studies or treatment, let's look more deeply at the powerful medicine at work. The medicine is the power within each of us to manifest our own healing by making a choice, both conscious and unconscious, to heal. The more we heal our trauma and release negative thoughts, the more deeply we can access the healing aspect of self. This is a superpower we humans have always had, but we forgot we had it. By using mind-over-matter techniques, people may be able to resolve wounds by letting go of old thoughts, beliefs, and attitudes.

For more information, check out the following books by Joe Dispenza, D.C.: *Breaking the Habit of Being Yourself: How to Lose Your Mind and Create a New One*, *Becoming Supernatural: How Common People Are Doing the Uncommon*, and *You Are the Placebo: Making Your Mind Matter*.

Understanding How We Are Wired

We can make the most of our abilities to make good decisions for ourselves and channel healing when we understand our responses, both conscious and unconscious, to our inner and outer environments. This overview explains the human nervous system as it relates to emotion, stress, and behavior, all of which affect both the progression of chronic Lyme disease and its treatment. As I discussed briefly in chapter 2, our nervous system is made up of the central nervous system and the peripheral nervous system. The central nervous system acts as the central processing unit of the body and is made up of the brain and the spinal cord. Moving out toward the periphery from the spinal column is the peripheral nervous system, which is divided into the somatic nervous system and the autonomic nervous system, further divided into the sympathetic nervous system, the parasympathetic nervous system, and the enteric nervous system. These all facilitate informational exchange, taking information in from the outside world, sending it to the central processing unit (brain), and then delivering a response. They are not separate but interdependent, providing us with the ability to experience a full life.

THE SYMPATHETIC NERVOUS SYSTEM

The sympathetic nervous system is about fight or flight. This mechanism makes us more vigilant and gives us the momentum to get ourselves out of danger. It helps the body and mind stay sharp in the moment so we can draw on bursts of energy to physically get through a dangerous situation. Our muscles receive more blood, which is shunted away from the gastrointestinal system, blood pressure rises, and our eyes open wider to improve visual acuity. A flood of the stress hormone cortisol can hyperstimulate the limbic system, an area of the brain related to fear response. If this response is triggered repeatedly, our brains may be rewired toward an outlook that life is not safe.

The limbic system lies deep in the cerebrum, close to the center of the brain; in this book, we are primarily interested in the amygdala and the hypothalamus. These areas of the brain are both involved in emotional response. The hypothalamus regulates the autonomic nervous system, which governs the stress response as well as many other functions in the body. The amygdala is specifically related to feelings of anger and fear. The amygdala is hyperstimulated in patients with a past history of trauma; they often have a fear response, even in nonthreatening situations. Trauma can be stored in multiple areas of the brain, which records sensations such as the taste, touch, smell, and sound associated with the events. The sense of smell has its own pathway related to memories, which is why odors can trigger memories and affect mood. The strong relationship to sensory experience is why people can have vivid memory recall or flashbacks related in which the sensory data are so real that a person feels as though she is in the situation all over again. Without proper support, this can be difficult to work through in a healthy way. The need to repress bad memories for self-protection often attracts people to numbing agents such as drugs or to avoidant behaviors that can distract them.

Lyme Rage

IN AN ARTICLE TITLED "Aggressiveness, Violence, Homicidality, Homicide, and Lyme Disease," Dr. Robert Bransfield addresses the increase in aggressive behaviors in those with tick-borne infections. I referenced another of Dr. Bransfield's articles, on Lyme disease and suicide risk, earlier in the chapter. In "Aggressiveness," he opens a dialogue about violent tendencies in those with neurological infections, specifically tick-borne disease. This is a topic of critical importance, as we face a rising epidemic in the United States, where many people with violent histories or mental illness have access to high-caliber weapons.

Thankfully, a majority of chronic Lyme patients have a level of self-control over violent actions; instead, they may turn aggression inward on themselves. None of my patients has committed criminal acts that warrant legal action or exhibited seriously violent behavior. However, my staff members and I have been the targets of unwarranted outbursts and physically threatening behaviors such as throwing items. These reactions are extreme, as the situations (such as having to wait for a task to be completed) would cause the average person only minor annoyance. Many chronic Lyme patients report increased aggravation, with feelings of rage toward family members, friends, coworkers, and the world. Some have reported violence in marriages, and patients have commented on thoughts of doing harm to others.

In a review of 1,000 charts, Dr. Bransfield found that a majority of the individuals studied did not manifest homicidal or extreme violent behavior until after they were confirmed with Lyme disease and coinfections. In my practice, I see aggression more frequently with the coinfection *Bartonella* than with confirmed Lyme disease. Among my patients, outbursts and harmful behaviors are reported more by parents of young Lyme disease patients, who hit siblings, throw items, threaten extreme violence, scream, and/or attack their parents. These behaviors are usually shocking to parents, as they have not witnessed these behaviors in their children before.

To explain the aggression, Dr. Bransfield points to hyperstimulation of aspects of the limbic system, such as the amygdala, due to brain inflammation, as well as inadequate serotonin levels. In addition, the areas of the brain that create empathy and a sense of community show reduced function, and this can override judgments that would inhibit violence. Other neurological factors are involved as well, but they are too complex to cover here.

The implications raised by aggressive tendencies in those with chronic Lyme disease and other tick-borne infections are troubling, as we see more cases of Lyme disease as the incidence of mass shootings rises. The good news is that a majority of patients, though they may feel more aggravated, would never participate in this type of violence. But the more we research this phenomenon, the better we will be at taking a preventive approach instead of waiting until after disaster has happened to look for a cause.[6]

THE PARASYMPATHETIC NERVOUS SYSTEM

The parasympathetic nervous system is associated with the impulse to "rest and digest." When we feel safe, our mind and heart are at peace and send messages to the rest of the body that it's safe. When we feel safe, our digestive system works like clockwork, blood flow is balanced throughout the body, heart rate is steady, we feel more joy and less pain, and we have improved immunity and balanced hormone function. In an ideal parasympathetic nervous system, the body is energy efficient and a person feels comfortable in his skin.

THE ENTERIC NERVOUS SYSTEM

The enteric nervous system is located in the lining of the gut. Sometimes called *the second brain*, this system has more than five hundred million neurons. It interacts with the other branches of the nervous system but can also function autonomously. The gastrointestinal tract interfaces with the outside world, as substances come in, and it communicates with the immune system, the microbiome, and the internal world of the central nervous system. It's also tied to our emotional state, intuitive decision making, motivation, and higher cognitive functioning.[7] There are several pathways between the gastrointestinal tract and the brain, including pathways that connect the sympathetic nervous system, adrenal glands, and immune system. Pathways also connect the amygdala, hypothalamus, and enteric nervous system referred to as the Gut-Brain Axis, which are both involved in our emotional responses, as discussed above. The three systems of the autonomic nervous system strive to work in harmony, in service to the body.

THE VAGUS NERVE

The vagus nerve, or the "wandering" nerve, is the tenth cranial nerve and one of the longest in the body. The vagus nerve communicates between the brain, heart, lungs, and the visceral organs to maintain calm, and it serves many functions, including assisting in swallowing and speech. It gives us the ability to sense taste at the back of the tongue and also acts as the sensor modifying behavior of the heart, lungs, and gastrointestinal tract. It lowers heart rate and blood pressure, decreases inflammation, and helps maintain healthy, deep, rhythmic breathing.

This nerve is all about feeling at peace, but it also innervates the sexual organs. Many patients complain of a lack of libido during illness, which is not only about hormones but also about the fact that they are not able to relax into their bodies due to stress and discomfort. With elevated levels of stress, anxiety, depression, and fear, the nervous system suppresses full sensation of pleasure. However, the vagus nerve also works in a way that is more akin to that of the sympathetic nervous system. This function is related to the polyvagal theory.

Neuroception and the Polyvagal Theory

Stephen Porges, Ph.D., explains the human stress response with the concept of neuroception and the polyvagal theory.[8] According to Dr. Porges, we are wired to survive but also need the ability to interact with one another so we can maintain healthy social groups, create loving relationships, sense when a situation is safe, and experience joy. Situations that feel unsafe are either obviously dangerous, requiring our bodies to mobilize rapidly, or are experienced internally like danger even when the outer experience appears safe. Dr. Porges calls this process of perception and evaluation *neuroception*. I would relate it to intuition, when our intuition is working in healthy state.

Dr. Porges uses as an example a child who responds to his mother with calm and openness so he can receive love. Yet, if a stranger initiated the same gesture that a mother does, the child would see it as dangerous and react emotionally with rejection. This sort of reaction happens in adults as well. Our nervous system reads situations as safe or unsafe, and we respond physically when we discern that a situation may not be safe, even if it is.

Neuroception can become problematic if we have underlying beliefs, emotional wounds, and negative thoughts created out of a trauma; that experience runs in the background, influencing our behavior in an unconscious way. The unconscious response can feel as if your mind is a horse running out of control, with your conscious mind trying calm down. The response can be hard to stop once it starts and comes in the form of increased heart rate, sweating, shaking, irrational emotional responses, dizziness, stimulation of the adrenal glands, and possible fainting.

This neuroceptive reaction can easily be out of sync with the actual situation if the person holds unconscious beliefs that others or the world are not safe. Clinically, I see the deepest wounds in those who experienced abuse from a parent, where one (or more) of the most important relationships in a person's life did not represent safety. When a child grows up feeling a continuous need to be on guard, the ramifications last over the course of a lifetime and leave few reserves to help the body heal from an infection such as chronic Lyme disease. Many of us may not have had an ideal childhood, but if most of our needs were met, we learned to cope. If, on the other hand, our bodies registered other people as unsafe, that reaction becomes hardwired into the nervous system in an unconscious way.

A person whose neuroceptive reaction is out of sync might label himself as having an anxiety disorder, depression, rage issues, or being fearful, and may admit that he can't help the reaction. Such an overreaction can also be related to scenarios such as being required to give a speech and feeling the physical sensations of stage fright. The neuroendocrine system is a powerful tool that gives us the ability to discern and react in a quick fashion, but it can be draining if it is triggered repeatedly.

Overly sensitive reactions also cause the quality of our social interactions to suffer. The neuroceptive system can work against us when we react from a place of emotional injury, in which unhealthy programs were built to defend us and help us survive. Initially, these served a purpose, but they later become a hindrance to healing. Because the danger response associated with neuroception can result from an outside perceived threat or an internal one, the inner sensation of pain, illness, and fevers can bring out intensely fearful reactions.

The polyvagal theory identifies two branches of the vagus, each with a different function, and addresses the relationship between experiences and the reactions of the vagus's parasympathetic system. According to the theory, there are three types of responses: mobilization, socialization, and immobilization.

Mobilization is triggered primarily by the sympathetic nervous system. This is the fight-or-flight impulse to escape real or perceived danger. Our senses become more acute, adrenaline pumps, energy is shunted to the body's muscles, the muscles of the face reflect fear, and our voice shows our stress. This is what happens when we are in protective mode, summoning our ability to defend ourselves while maintaining sharpened senses.

Socialization, or the social engagement system, involves the rest-and-digest impulse and is the primary function of the parasympathetic nervous system. Its function is to calm the heart, regulate digestion, inhibit the adrenals from expressing stress hormones, and show welcoming facial expressions. When we are in this mode, our voice is calm, and we create healthy social interactions. The social engagement system is regulated by the parasympathetic ventral vagal complex.

The third response, immobilization, is mediated by the vagal nerve as part of the parasympathetic dorsal vagal complex. This is a primitive response. The reaction involves playing dead physically, mentally, or emotionally; it can literally create a freeze response, leading to reduced heart rate, unresponsive facial expression, passing out, and a reduced ability to hear clearly or communicate. Emotions are flat; we shut down. We behave like a deer in the headlights or a small animal that ceases all movement instead of running away.

These three responses are all biological solutions created by the body to survive based on information from past experiences. Why is it so important that the chronic Lyme disease community understand these responses? If wiring makes your nervous system overrespond or underrespond to a stressor, your ability to move through the treatment process will be impaired. An out-of-proportion response to stress may be one reason that some people recover easily from tick-borne disease while others have a long and difficult road.

Many factors, known and unknown, contribute to this variability in recovery, and when we look into unconscious biological wiring, our goal is to learn to rewire ourselves for optimal health. Instead of seeing the body as a betrayer holding on to illness, we can perceive it as a benevolent system with a strong sense of protection. With mindfulness techniques and counseling, we can learn to rewire these responses.

Since Dr. Porges brought his theory forward in the early 1990s, it has been tested in many ways to study its implications for mental health, physical illness, and other facets of human health. All three states—mobilization, socialization, and immobilization—have a purpose, but they need to be in balance to create resilience in the face of stressors. The freeze response, or immobilization, happens when the other two systems are not able to provide signals strong enough to override the lower neurological responses.

How can we strengthen our resilience and enhance a healthy neurological response? An article published in *Frontiers in Human Neuroscience* titled "Yoga Therapy and Polyvagal Theory: The Convergence of Traditional Wisdom and Contemporary Neuroscience for Self-Regulation and Resilience" detailed a method of healing that views the body from top-down and bottom-up regulatory processes. Top-down processes are related to meditation and mindfulness practices that rewire our attention and intention. As we rewire our minds for calm, we can improve our immune system, downregulate our fight-or-flight response, and decrease inflammation. Bottom-up processes use body movement (e.g, yoga or Qigong) and biofield therapies (e.g., Reiki). These practices can improve the function of the digestive system, musculoskeletal system, cardiovascular system, and neurological processes. Thinking in terms of healing from a bidirectional model improves our resilience with time and commitment to contemplative practices.

Interoception: Going Inward

With the use of meditation, yoga, Qigong, energy healing, talk therapy, and many other mind-body-spirit modalities, we can improve our sense of interoception.[9] Interoception is the ability to be more in tune and aware of the responses of our bodies, allowing us to step into witness mode and choose our response with more empowered intention. Sensations that create pain, whether expected or unexpected, can increase anxiety, and this is more likely to create more pain. Enhancing interoception creates greater presence in the moment and improves our ability to craft a better outcome. It involves bringing our awareness back to our own needs, our own bodies, and our emotions.

Meditation can open us up to the information behind the curtain of the unconscious mind.

Contemplative practices are the best way to enhance interoception, and many options are available. The option you choose matters less than the fact that you are working in conjunction with others to provide safe space to do this work and learning applicable tools you can use in individual practice. Find a meditation style or mindfulness practice you are interested in—one which will motivate you to show up. The profound aspects of mindfulness, contemplation, and therapeutic movement modalities are in the act of doing them. Each person gets what she needs from the practice in the exact time she needs to experience it. Your ego is not in charge of the outcome, but it is in charge of showing up to be witness to the possibilities.

Making Time to Feel

Creating space and time is important to any form of contemplative or mindfulness practice. As we start to tune in, we may experience sensations that are not easy to be with. If we have not listened to our mind-body in a long time, the body may have accumulated information and may be waiting for permission to reveal it. Just as we detoxify the body of physical substances, we also need to detoxify emotionally and mentally. Mental-emotional clutter can accumulate, adding to our stress, low immunity, and physical pain with increased inflammation, undesired moods, and poor concentration. This is more likely to happen if you were raised in an environment in which showing emotion was considered a weakness or a liability.

Our conscious mind is aware of such a small part of our experience at any given time, but meditation can open us up to the information behind the curtain of the unconscious mind. Our inner critic, also referred to as the *pain body*, can emerge; it is the part of us that holds feelings of lack, resentment, inferiority, anger, grief, shame, trauma, and others that enhance pain rooted in fear.

Eckhart Tolle, a modern-day spiritual teacher, coined the term the *pain body*. While it sounds ominous, it is the accumulated stagnant energies in a subtle body of judgment, self-loathing, and other unloving thoughts that can be felt emotionally and physically. Tolle also alludes to the fact that we can have an attachment to our pain body, which can be related to a victim mentality, an inability to forgive, and difficulty taking personal responsibility. As you open up to listening, it's natural to experience pent-up emotions such as sadness, anger, victimhood, and overwhelm; and these can be aligned with areas of discomfort in the body. When energy can't find a solution or resolution, it is stored in the body. Unresolved mental, emotional, or physical pain is retained by the ego mind, which repeats the pattern of pain through our reactions again and again.

Bring Yourself into the Now Moment

When we have unresolved trauma, we are straddling the past and projecting into the future. This means it is more difficult to feel at home in our body in the present moment. When we project into the future, we cultivate anxiety by creating stories about what will happen in the future. Usually, we rely on catastrophic thinking. The mind is creative, and can come up with all sorts of unbelievable movie-of-the-week outcomes. The more we think these thoughts, the more our brains reinforce them, looping over and over again. One of these loops can be, "I'm never going to be well again."

In many cultures, it's common to make time to cry or for other emotional release. I recommend that you take time on regular basis to sit, stand, or lie down in a sacred space you have created. Ideally, this is a place where you won't be interrupted. Simply make the statement, in your mind or out loud, "I *am* here and available to release feelings or sensations that are beneficial for healing." Then breathe and allow feelings to surface. Nothing may happen initially if you are used to swallowing your feelings as a survival mechanism. This process creates a space to allow air out of the balloon slowly, with intention, so it does not build up.

You may start to feel emotions rise through your body as a somatic experience of sensation, with muscles tensing and relaxing. This is normal as emotions move out of the tissues and subtle body and detox gets under way. If the emotions start to feel unsafe or overwhelming, pull back. Bring your awareness back a few steps. This practice is not about forcing the emotions to move but about allowing the intelligence of the body-mind to work the energy through the system. If you have a history of traumatic memories, these may resurface if they are trapped. In this case, it's advisable to work with a counselor to help you process the emotions that emerge.

Self-care, such as establishing regular sleep patterns and eating healthily, is also very important at this time. Deep emotional work is best partnered with yoga, Qigong, Tai Chi, exercise, massage, and/or sauna to allow energy to continue to be released in a healthy way. These exercises also let you participate in nurturing yourself, which fosters compassion for self. Trauma work is a practice to undertake when you have social support and can authentically share the emotions that arise, integrating healing.

Contemplative practices that can be modified to fit anyone's capabilities include:

- **Meditation, daily or several times per week:** You can do guided meditations, where you listen to others take you on a journey, or repeat prayer/mantra statements to focus on. You can also do moving meditation (hiking or dancing) or just be with your breath in solitude. Meditation is a time to detoxify your mind of thoughts that have accumulated from stress responses to inner and outer experiences. The eventual goal is to just be with yourself, your breath, and your thoughts and to learn to listen internally without outside interaction. Just as we detox the physical body, we must detox the mental body, pain body, and emotional body. Everyone can meditate: You just need to keep showing up to the practice, have a comfortable place to be, and keep breathing. Start with ten to fifteen minutes per day.

- **Creation of a sacred space:** Find a place of solitude at home, at work, or outside (garden, ocean, hiking trail, bench in a park). It could even be a chair in the house. This is just a place where you can sit, signaling that you are in need of time to be quiet with your thoughts. The intention and the physiological response to being in the space are both vital. Setting aside a special place is rooted in ritual and is part of many different spiritual and mindfulness practices that change the frequency of the brain to a calmer state. Just by being in the space—with certain smells, colors, pictures, furniture, sacred objects, stones or crystals, or books that have meaning for you—you can instantaneously improve your state of mind. This can become your primary space for meditation or simply a place to be creative.

- **Movement, with yoga/Qigong/Tai Chi/walking/running:** As we move our bodies with intention and purpose, we move stagnant energy that accumulates in muscles, nerves, lymphatic vessels, digestive tract, and energetic circulatory systems. This improves the mind-body connection as well as strengthens the body; movement can reduce pain and enhance mood through expression of healthy neurotransmitters. Initially, you may experience growing pains, as you improve your endurance. Most of the movements prescribed can be done while sitting or lying down, just moving the limbs, or you can fully engage with your whole body. Use your own judgment to discern the best starting point because no one knows you better than you; but do not be afraid to push out of your comfort zone. Mild to moderate discomfort is where change will happen. But I do not recommend any unnecessary suffering in any way.

In Summary

I have seen patients change deeply when chronic Lyme disease goes into remission. Often, surmounting their challenges leaves them with a deeper understanding of what they want to do, and new talents emerge. One patient cultivated the ability to paint, even though she'd previously been so neuro-logically compromised she could barely speak, walk normally, or pay attention during our visits. It took her a few years to recover, but she is now selling her fantastic pieces. Another patient had been overextended, caring for everyone else to the detriment of her own health. She made the decision to choose herself by creating better boundaries with others for the sake of her own well-being. As soon as she did, something changed in her disease process, and she quickly gained more energy, became more gregarious, and determined to get well. She had been losing weight, felt terrible pain, and was neurologically compromised, but her health steadily improved when she made herself a priority.

Others have felt motivated to create social justice for those dealing with Lyme disease, creating fund-raising and support groups. Going through the recovery process enables individuals to take the lessons into their work life, especially those in the health care field. Most doctors who are outspoken about tick-borne infections have gone through their own health crisis with Lyme disease, which focuses their attention toward advocacy, research, and education. I include myself among these; I had been treating Lyme disease for several years before discovering I also was infected.

Understanding underlying issues in the psyche can greatly help a growing population of chronically ill people with tick-borne infection. Let's change the focus from chronic Lyme disease as a fictional illness or shameful diagnosis to one that has potential for healing. The well-known Sufi mystic and poet Rumi says, "The wound is where the light enters you." Let's allow this to happen.

Let's acknowledge our wounds so we can start to heal them, regain health, empower ourselves, and move through the world with ease. This must start with allowing the energy around the situation to change. Chronic illness can be painful and humbling, but it is the best medicine for healing your life once you set up a process and support network to help you. If you have been diagnosed with psychosomatic illness, say, "Thank you. Yes, I do." Your mind and body are not separate and never have been. Science is starting to finally acknowledge this aspect of medicine, and this new attitude will eventually trickle down into the inner workings of the average doctor's office.

CHAPTER 11

ENERGY MEDICINE: NURTURING OUR FUTURE SELVES

Medications are external supports intended to improve the health of the body. As much as we try to find answers to illness and infection in a bottle or a machine, we should not ignore the power of the individual to heal from within. This power has just barely been tapped into by the majority of the population. For instance, researchers have discovered that IL-6—an inflammation marker commonly elevated in the brains of those who commit acts of self-harm—can be decreased by feelings of "awe," experienced in states of joy, bliss, contentment, or relaxation.[1]

Energy medicine is a difficult topic to delve into. It's a subject that strikes a chord in people—it either resonates or brings out skepticism. There are so many opportunities to receive energy healing as a form of treatment—now more than ever before. New healing centers are opening up, and energy therapies are being integrated into medical practices, counseling centers, hospitals, and education facilities. The corporate world, too, has begun to also incorporate energy medicine by encouraging mindfulness practices during the workday to improve employees' mental focus and morale.

In this chapter, I discuss my own journey into the energy medicine world, offer scientific validation of energy therapies, and offer an overview of shamanism, Reiki, and other energy medicine, showing the benefits of incorporating them into your Lyme disease treatment plan.

My Story

Many patients ask how I got into energy medicine. I have always been intrigued by the science behind the mind-body connection. My interest started at the age of nine or ten with a fascination of accounts of near-death experiences, most likely propelled by the death of my mother when I was seven. Like many children, I was very sensitive, but I learned to suppress the things I somehow knew, my deep feelings of empathy for others, and the things I saw and heard that I could not explain. I also found it difficult to relax into these experiences while feeling deep grief in the early years of my life. The mystical experiences also scared me. I was not taught how to be in harmony with them, so I felt overwhelmed. Throughout most of my childhood and young adulthood, I suffered intense social anxiety and was painfully shy. I suppressed a lot of myself and did not really embrace who I was until I experienced a Kundalini awakening in my mid-thirties.

This awakening started with a profound experience during a meditation where I left my body and expanded in a bliss state, hearing clearly the statement, "Remember who you are." I took days to return to normal. A few weeks later, the feeling came back even stronger, with an intense sensation shooting up my spine, waking me out of sleep. I went through a difficult time trying to understand the overwhelming number of physical, mental, emotional, and spiritual experiences that were happening simultaneously. This went on for many months.

I was experiencing something Stan Grof, M.D., Ph.D., researcher and author, refers to as a *spiritual emergency* or *psychospiritual crisis*. A psycho-spiritual crisis is one in which a person's self-concept and place in the world completely shift after a spontaneous mystical experience. This is a transformational experience, evolutionary and healing, though it was hard to see it like that while deep in it. Many people have gone through this process or are going through it now.

It was difficult to maintain my daily life of medical practice and motherhood. Some days, I was not functional at all and hid away, desperately wanting solitude. Caroline Myss, a well-known medical intuitive and author, gave a great lecture titled "Spiritual Madness," in which she discussed the phenomenon of energy openings in the modern world. Historically, when people experienced spiritual events like the one that happened to me, they would have gone to a monastery, abbey, or ashram to find solitude. It is much more difficult in the modern world to find space for solitude while maintaining a routine life.

Initially, I investigated both physical and psychological reasons for my experience. I had spinal taps, CT scans, blood work, and MRIs. I was at first concerned that I had had a stroke or a brain injury from the Lyme disease. I was having visions, receiving auditory information, and having physical sensations, pain, and body movements with spontaneous yoga postures, which frightened me. At the same time, I knew I was moving through something that was ultimately benevolent in nature. I consulted with medical practitioners, priests, psychologists, and energy healers and read as much as I could to figure out how to make it stop. But it didn't stop, so I surrendered to the process.

It took me a while to understand I was having a mystical, physical, emotional, and psychological experience all at the same time. With the help of a knowledgeable circle of support, I was able to put myself back together with a new transpersonal understanding and healing abilities. Since this shift, I devour books on energy healing and have attended multiple trainings in energy-healing modalities for my own benefit and so I can integrate them into my medical practice.

I'm a lifelong student and a work in progress. I hope this personal revelation is helpful to others in some way. It's difficult to convey the magnitude of these experiences, as most people who have had them will tell you. Once you try to explain the mystery, it loses potency and gets watered down. I know this chapter is a radical departure from the rest of the book, but it is near and dear to my heart as well as big part of my medical practice.

Working with an Energy Medicine Provider

Lyme disease treatments involving energy-healing modalities are becoming more and more common, among them color therapy that exposes the blood to different colors in the light spectrum, magnetic therapies that change the movement of ions in the body, sound therapy with crystal healing bowls that emit healing frequencies, medical intuition, shamanic healing, healing with intention, different forms of yoga, flower essences, homeopathy, meditation, and Reiki. In addition, there are rife machines, which introduce healing frequencies through special amplifiers and coils placed on the body, as well as machines that can test the body's reactions to different remedies to find the most auspicious combination for healing. The motivation in seeking out these therapies with an open mind is a desire to heal.

When you are working with a practitioner in an energy session, you are learning—and not only what can be read or spoken. Energy work is an education of listening and experiential learning for all involved. A session is a time and place to learn how to acknowledge emotions and physical sensations while working with the subtle states of energy. Your energy is transformed by the space created between you, the practitioner, and universal energy. There is infinite potential for change. You may need just one appointment with an energy-healing practitioner to set you on the path to healing. Others, myself included, may have multiple sessions, peeling away layers over time in a learn-as-you-go method taken at your own pace.

The motivation in seeking out these therapies with an open mind is a desire to heal.

As I work with patients in energy-healing sessions, which are distinct from standard medical office visits, I use an amalgamation of the modalities I've studied over the years. This results in a unique experience each time. I'm very kinesthetic, experiencing energy in my physical body. I have an inner physical knowledge of where to place my hands over a patient's body and use a blend of sight, sound, and touch as needed to provide information that is helpful for the patient. Rather than doing the healing, I act as the conduit for the energy flow that assists the process. Each meeting is different and depends on the needs of the individual seeking help and what is best for her at the time of the visit. I strive to create a safe space, work with integrity, and never take away a patient's personal power.

Patients have shared amazing stories of synchronicities, clarity of thought, a better relationship with their own bodies, beautiful mystical experiences, beneficial dreams, profound changes in family dynamics, and self-empowerment. Energy healing can be done in conjunction with medications—there is no need to choose one over the other—and it embraces and honors any tradition or belief system. These sessions can help to reduce Herxheimer reactions, improve coping skills, induce deeper healing of past trauma, aid in detoxification, calm the nervous system, and offer many other benefits.

You might see a wide variety of costs associated with energy treatments as well as promises of a cure. This type of treatment requires more discernment from consumers, who must consider legitimate business practices and the ethics of energy healing—patients need to be savvy about navigating this world without becoming mesmerized by the magic and mystery. Always ask about a practitioner's training, methods, and how he views his role. A practitioner who cultivates fear to create more drama is not going to be a healthy choice; energy healing requires that a provider be authentic without overanalyzing the information, fortune telling, or disempowering the client by claiming superiority.

Where Science and Spirit Meet

The field of quantum physics offers a bridge between material reality, such as our bodies, and a reflection of universal energy. Albert Einstein once referred to the ability of one particle to communicate directly with another at a great distance as a "spooky" event; known as *quantum entanglement*, this has now gone beyond theory and is a proven physical phenomenon. Plants can compute using quantum mechanics during photosynthesis. They preferentially absorb the most beneficial color particles in the light spectrum, which move through the leaf with a single photon particle simultaneously in more than one place at a time. The plant does this for survival, finding the most efficient pathway for light to reach it destination, becoming 100 percent energy efficient.[2]

In peer-reviewed research, energy healing modalities are referred to as *biofield therapies*, defined as "gentle, noninvasive therapies that work in the human energy field." The term *biofield* was introduced at a conference of the U.S. National Institutes of Health in 1992. Biofield therapies have since branched into various medical applications, including biofield physiology, in which energy fields code information and provide instructions that influence biological systems, such as the magnetic fields generated by the heart cells.[3]

Biofield therapies cover a wide variety of modalities, including Qigong, yoga, hands-on healing, power of prayer (intention), acupuncture, the external use of magnets, flower essences, homeopathy, Pranic healing, shamanic healing, and many others. A study published in the journal *Alternative Therapies in Health and Medicine* reported that biofield therapies reduced pain and tenderness in the body while improving depression in patients diagnosed with fibromyalgia to a degree that allowed a majority of participants to reduce their medication use.[4] Therapeutic touch is recognized in hospital settings, where it's now common to have Reiki practitioners work with patients to reduce stress and improve recovery rates. In the 2012 National Health Interview Survey conducted by the U.S. Centers for Disease Control, 3.7 million people replied yes when asked if they had ever seen an energy-healing practitioner.[5] I would guess that this number is even higher now, with chronic disease on the rise creating a trend toward alternative therapies driving the marketplace.

As technology has improved, we are able to prove the existence of the auric field or light fields radiating from all living beings, which are referred to as *biophotons*. Biophotons are ultraweak photonic light emitted from biological systems as luminescence; they are not related to heat but change based on stress on the living system. Fluctuations in biophoton emissions have been found in relationship to cerebral blood flow and energy metabolism in the brain. Understanding their function could lead us to ways to observe imbalances medically before they manifest as physical illness.

Biophotons were first discussed by Alexander Gurwitsch, who believed that fields of energy governed physical development. He called these *morphogenetic fields* and posited that cells interact with each other to develop specific organ systems or draw together to complete a task. This idea was later expanded by physicist Fritz-Albert Popp, Ph.D., who revived the concept after using more advanced technology to witness light emanating from tissues.

Accessing the Collective Unconscious for Healing

Rupert Sheldrake, Ph.D., a cell biologist and author of several books and articles, hypothesized the concept of *morphic resonance fields,* shared fields of information that hold inherent memories. A morphic resonance field allows an underlying nonverbal understanding of a collective unconscious shared by members of a species or group.

The *collective unconscious,* a term coined by one of the fathers of modern psychology, Carl Jung, is data that informs the physical world using archetypes, or universal patterns and images. Think of it like a spiritual Internet. Our minds are able to respond and change based on data that are part of our larger cultural knowledge base, even though we might look at something and feel we have no understanding of it—it's what we might think of as instinct or as recognition of a universal symbol.

The concept of archetypes was best illustrated to me through a healing method I studied called the Mora Technique 7 Layers of the Heart, developed by shamanic practitioner Esther Mora, D.D., D.MT. It involves using archetypal images, which can include mathematical equations rooted in physics, binary code sequences, chemical structures of medicinal plants, sacred geometry, and many others. The higher aspect of the mind connected with the collective unconscious understands how to use the data to improve mental, emotional, and physical balance. It begs the question: Do we always need to take medications into the body to create change? Can we heal the physical body instead by accessing the collective unconscious or morphic fields? This is fascinating stuff—and it means we have more healing power within than we realize.

Quantum Dosing of Nutraceuticals

IN CERTAIN PRACTICES, SUCH AS SHAMANISM, everything is alive with consciousness and spirit, including plants. Working with the energy fields of consciousness can enhance the healing potential of plant-based medicine by working with intention to ask for healing from the consciousness of the plant.

I typically have on hand an herbal combination in capsule form to support the adrenal glands, with ashwagandha, licorice root, holy basil, and rhodiola. I use these herbs as an example; you can use whatever you have at home, as long as it is plant based. Take one or two pills in your left hand (you may feel a pull to place them in your right hand, which also works). Before you swallow the medication, sit with the capsules in your hand. Ask for the plant intelligence or its archetype to work with you to allow healing to go where it is most needed within. Then thank it for its assistance.

You may feel movement, heat, and tingling in your mid-back, where the adrenals are located. If you don't feel anything, it does not mean the intention-setting is not working, but I know it makes it easier to connect with the process if you have some confirmation. You can then take the pill internally. I would caution you to use this method only with homeopathic remedies, flower essences, nutrients, and other forms of plant medicine found in the natural world. Don't try this with pharmaceuticals, though you can ask the body to resonate with any medication before you swallow it, to help create balance. Plants are our greatest medicine, teachers, and food resources on the planet. Without them, we could not survive. If you want to know more about this topic, look for one of the many books referencing plant spirit medicine, or consult the HeartMath Institute for its research on plant intelligence with the "Interconnectivity Tree Research Project."

Our Energy Anatomy

Energy anatomy is a more significant part of our lives than we acknowledge. Crediting its role and learning to work with it is a game changer for our health, communication, emotional responses, cognition, and quality of life. One of the most ancient forms of medicine, now common around the world, acupuncture works within the subtle energy field of the body's meridians, mapped out by healers and doctors over centuries. Meridians are aligned with other aspects of energy anatomy, the chakra system and etheric/auric energy fields.

It's helpful to have a basic understanding of our energy anatomy. There are many different schools of thought, which use different terminology. The specific layers of energy radiate from the body—you can think of these like the layers of a Russian nesting doll. You keep removing the outer layers until you find the physical body at the center. The energy anatomy briefly discussed here are the chakras, the meridians, and the etheric body.

Commonly referred to as *Prana* or *Qi* (Chi), the energy breathes in and out, informing our cells and DNA as it moves through a refined mesh and duct system aligned with organ systems. The areas in which this energy is concentrated are referred to as *chakras*, now a fairly familiar concept in our Western vernacular. The term *chakra* refers to a spinning wheel of energy concentrated at specific points in the body. The seven major chakras are aligned with the glandular system along the spinal column, although there are many more minor ones. Each chakra has a particular function, movement, sound, color, relationship with our mental/emotional body, ancestral connection, immunity, and soul life. Eastern medicine modalities have a more integrated approach to the energy meridians and medicine than Westernized medical practices do. Chakras have been mapped out over centuries, and these lines of force are used by acupuncturists to restore flow of our energy within the etheric body, which is not separate from other aspects of energy anatomy.

The etheric body sits right against the physical body, with intricately woven threads or lines of force communicating directly with our cellular structure as well as receiving outer energy information. The etheric body holds our memories and ancestral information. For instance, phantom limb sensations experienced by those who have lost an arm or leg are related to the etheric body. The continued awareness of the limb and sensations in the absence of the physical body part is due to the energetic limb still being present and experienced by the nervous system through the etheric blueprint.

Plants, minerals, or animals, when exposed to high-voltage electric field energy, emit a light energy residue. This is well documented with Kirlian photography, discovered by Russian scientist Semyon Kirlian in 1938. When parts of plants are removed, for example, the image of the original physical form remains in subsequent photos. This represents visual proof of what amputees experience physically, the presence of the etheric energy map, which underlies physical structure and is still associated with the structure even though physical parts are missing.

Energy flows into the etheric field, which then informs our physical cells and affects the body's response, becoming part of our physical experience. If the etheric body is storing unhealthy energy from electromagnetic smog put out by cell phones, emotional wounds, ancestral trauma, or individual trauma, or is holding any data that do not resonate with healing, the physical body's quality of life is affected, making it more susceptible to disease. If the quality of life in the body is poor, the mental/emotional state of the person is affected, perpetuating a vicious cycle. All energy modalities, at their core, attempt to remove blockages to energy flow, whether the obstruction is rooted in mental/emotional blocks, toxic body burden, microbial interactions, or nutritional imbalances. Once flow is reestablished, the body can more readily remove toxins, create balance with microbes in the body, reduce stress, and restore proper function for improved quality of life.

For a deeper dialogue on energy anatomy, I suggest reading Barbara Ann Brennan's book *Hands of Light: A Guide to Healing Through the Human Energy Field* or Caroline Myss's *Anatomy of the Spirit: The Seven Stages of Power and Healing.*

Creating a New Relationship with Microbes

The Gaia hypothesis, developed by scientists James Lovelock, Ph.D., D.Sc., and Lynn Margulis, Ph.D., in 1972, states that Earth is an evolving, interconnected living system that is continually finding solutions to maintain homeostasis. Microbes inhabited the planet 2.1 billion years before there were any signs of animal or plant life,[6] and the bacterium that causes Lyme disease has been shown by genetic sequencing to have been in the United States between twenty thousand and sixty thousand years ago.

Dr. Margulis, a biologist, researcher, and author, also coined the term *holobiont* to describe the relationship of the human, animal, or plant to its microorganisms. Years later, the name *hologenome* was brought forth by scientists Eugene Rosenberg, Ph.D., and Ilana Zilber-Rosenberg, Ph.D.[7] The hologenome is made up of the total genes of the host and all its symbiotic microbes. These are in relationship passed from generation to generation as well as transmitted horizontally via other humans, ticks, animals, and the environment (through water, air, and soil). There can be subtle or more dramatic changes in the hologenome, depending on what's required for survival. The key to our adaptability on Earth is our interrelationship with microbes because of the ability of their genomes to change more rapidly than the human genome does. Thus, microbes are our informers and our problem solvers.

Lyme disease is referred to as the *disease of the soul* in a healing modality called *microbioenergetics*, developed by Miguel Ojeda Rios, M.D.

Microbioenergetics is an amalgam of microbiology, embryology, neurology, epigenetics, bioenergetics, New Germanic Medicine, Biomagnetic Pair Therapy (application of magnets to change pH in body to resolve physical imbalances), psychology, Family Constellation Work, muscle testing, and more. This modality is a dynamic, ever-evolving practice that is too immense to cover in detail here. There are many parallels with the work of Dietrich Klinghardt, M.D., Ph.D., and his applied psychoneurobiology courses through the Klinghardt Academy. Both doctors have been profoundly helpful in expanding my approach to the complexities of diseases such as Lyme disease by offering a road map to help find the core of the individual's connection with his energy field and the disease causing suffering.

Changing your relationship with the microbe and learning to be in harmony with it starts by changing your relationship with yourself.

Microbioenergetics is about finding a way to understand where the human being and the microbe meet within the body from an emotional perspective; then trying to understand how this interaction is fostering illness in the individual. Changing your relationship with the microbe and learning to be in harmony with it starts by changing your relationship with yourself. This is related to the Law of Attraction or Law of Mirroring, which looks at what inside us attracts that which is outside of us, creating an energetic resonance. If something resonates with us, we create a relationship with it. Once that resonance is gone, the relationship has no purpose anymore and it changes. Why is the microbe making a home in us? What does it have to teach us? As we go deeper into these questions, we may find past traumas, emotions, and beliefs that are in alignment with illness.

Microbioenergetics uses the art of asking questions with applied kinesiology to get direct information from the higher intelligence of the mind-body connection. This is done by asking yes or no questions, then interpreting changes in leg length, usually in the right leg; this is information sourced from a deeper interpersonal knowledge, associated with the right brain rather than the analytical left brain. When working with the higher intelligence of the body aligned with the universal energy field, we can find answers unfettered by our doubts and personal filters.

The main goal is to identify a personal conflict, conscious or unconscious, that is aligned with a particular microbe. Conflicts are rooted in primal needs such as those for food, land, shelter, safety, love, and water. Conflicts in the modern world may center on lack of job, lack of love, or loss of a home. However, the core aspect of these conflicts are rooted in primal survival

Lyme disease has the ability to poke you emotionally and root out feelings you had stored away for self-protection.

needs. Once this information is brought to the surface, we have an opportunity to change the relationship with the microbe by healing our inner wounds, by merely bringing inner information into the awareness of the conscious mind, which then prompts a release from the body. This release can be mental, emotional, physical, or at the soul level.

When a patient has failed multiple treatment regimens, I commonly ask patients in my initial microbioenergetics session, "Do you want to be well?" When I ask this, the person looks at me with a raised brow and says of course they want to be well. Why else would they be here, participating in this process? Then I ask the body, and the body says, NO. Shock shows on the patient's face, as she doesn't understand how that could be. We have more power than we acknowledge to alter the course of our biology. If a patient has unconscious feelings of inadequacy, undeservedness, punishment, guilt, or shame, or holds beliefs handed down through generations, her unconscious choice has a profound impact on her health. This could be why the multiple therapies she has tried have failed. Rather than the medicine, her unconscious choice may be dictating the course of the disease. Once this belief is brought to light, the biological energy aligned with it changes and is no longer supported. Then the biology changes, based on the new belief, and is more receptive to healing. This is just one example of a potential reason that recovery from Lyme disease can be difficult.

To circle back to Lyme disease as a disease of the soul, it seems this intelligent microbe could have the job of collective catalyst, bringing forth inner fears so we can experience the gift of releasing them. These are deeper fears carried within societies, communities, and cultures. Lyme disease has a way of shining a spotlight on the shadows buried within. I always found it interesting that one of the cardinal homeopathic remedies for Lyme disease is aurum (gold), the most coveted illuminated metal on the planet. Aurum is also a remedy for dark thoughts and feelings.

Your emotions can become erratic not only due to neuroinflammation but also because of hidden feelings such as repressed anger, sadness, grief, shame, and fear. Your ability to trust others, to feel safe, and to have faith in your body will be triggered and tested during the process of recovery. Lyme disease has the ability to poke you emotionally and root out feelings you had stored away for self-protection. These stored emotions can become toxic and work against you if they are not resolved.

Reconnecting with Our Personal Power: Shamanism

Energy-healing modalities can help us expand self-knowledge, find personal power in a disempowering situation, and heal not just from physical complaints but from psychological stressors as well. Energy medicine also is a way to reorient our relationship with our bodies, the environment, and our family dynamics. It provides an opportunity to go inward and search for our own unique answers to our health crises, in conjunction with external medications. The goal of these modalities is to remove impediments to health so the body can do what it knows how to do—return to balance, create deeper states of peace and hope, and enhance personal power. Energy-healing modalities can make healing more efficient but are not meant to take the place of other medical interventions; instead, they can work alongside any path a patient takes on his personal healing journey.

I have observed enough individuals moving through chronic Lyme disease to notice a pattern in which the ability to retain old suffering is no longer possible. If a person continues to resist her pain and suffering, the illness manifests on a grander scale. These shadows can create tension within, leading to disease. Shamanic healing arts offer another way to relieve this tension, to let go of repressed energy and bring harmony into areas of discord. The difficulty with any healing journey is finding patience with the process and being able to trust the information given in a mystical experience, which is usually given in metaphor, either through direct experience or through a practitioner tuning in to get information on behalf of another.

Shamanism has been around for tens of thousands of years, but its traditions were historically kept closed, shared only by word of mouth with those initiated into the practice. Shamanism has traditionally been embraced by cultures that feel a deep sense of connection to the planet and their community, and to the plant, mineral, and animal kingdoms. One could argue that this connection has been lost in the modern Westernized world, leaving a sense of separation from nature. In shamanic practice, everything has consciousness, and everything is connected. Sentient beings include plants, minerals, microbes, the elements, the animal kingdom, and Earth herself.

A shaman is one who can walk between worlds, with one foot in ordinary reality and the other in nonordinary reality, accessed in deep states of meditative journey. Shamanic practitioners learn techniques to access nonordinary reality through the power of focus, intention, will, and prayer, which cultivate deeper meditative states. A spiritual practice rather than a religion, shamanism can be woven into any tradition or belief system. It's also a partnership with helping spirits and higher intelligence as the guiding force. This idea of being in service is part of almost every spiritual practice, cross-culturally.

Shamans are typically initiated through a crisis; this can be a health crisis, a near-death experience, or a mental-emotional crisis, or it can be a spontaneous opening to nonordinary realms through meditative practices. The process of moving through tick-borne infection can be a form of initiation. Initiation is the process of walking through a painful trial and coming out on the other side stronger and more spiritually mature.

Healers use common shamanic practices referred to as *shamanic journeying* and *shamanic ceremony*. We can all cultivate these skills. The goal is to become the "hollow bone"—essentially, a conduit—by clearing your mind of daily mundane thoughts and allowing higher information to come through. Shamanic practitioners usually use a drum, rattle, or dance to encourage thoughts to fall away and to permit deeper listening. As you become more skilled in the practice, you learn to get into a receptive state much more quickly.

Those who practice shamanism journey on behalf of themselves, another individual, a group, or the land to access healing information; but shamanism is also is a way of connecting with our ancestral lineage so that we can heal family patterns—for our own benefit but also for our descendants. The role of the client receiving healing is to remain receptive and calm. The role of the shamanic practitioner is not to analyze data but to allow information to be relayed authentically in a way that cultivates a healthy outcome. It's a dynamic creative practice with many applications and methods, always changing to stay relevant in a given culture and time. Shamanic methods are used in medicine, psychology, sociology, and in areas of commerce. These practices and tools are accessible because individuals have been able to meld traditions of shamanism with Western conventions.

My motivation in discussing shamanism is to foreground its relevance to our health care system, where illness has many causes, including a loss of power. Diseases are treated in the body with medications, but if the core cause is a broader issue, finding profound levels of healing may be challenging. Shamanism is not about guaranteeing a miracle, but it can produce profound shifts that improve health. Reconnecting with the sacred and working with the energy available in the universe for healing is the primary motivation in shamanic practice. It's about self-care, personal responsibility, compassion, and connection with all beings as a unified system. It is not a new way of being but rather a remembering of who we are.

Shamanism aligns beautifully with the tenets of naturopathic medicine, in which the doctor is teacher and helps channel the healing power of nature. Many shamanic teachers I have worked with have trained with the Foundation for Shamanic Studies, founded by the late Michael Harner, Ph.D. His books *The Way of the Shaman* and *Cave and Cosmos: Shamanic Encounters with Another Reality* are excellent resources for exploring shamanic healing practice further. I never had the opportunity to meet Dr. Harner, but I'm grateful for his work in bringing shamanism into Western culture. Another fantastic resource are the books of one of my teachers, Sandra Ingerman: *Shamanic Journeying: A Beginner's Guide*, *Walking in Light: The Everyday Empowerment of a Shamanic Life*, and *Medicine for the Earth: How to Transform Personal and Environmental Toxins*. There are many different lineages in shamanic practice, with teachers around the world; there are also plentiful opportunities for online learning.

Reiki

Reiki is a form of healing that originated in Japan. *Rei* means "higher power" and *Ki* means "life force." Thus, Reiki is the laying on of hands, typically via hovering of hands with intention: It's working with the intention and source energy that moves through all beings. Reiki connects us directly with universal energy flow. Those attuned to Reiki set the intention to allow the life force to flow where healing is needed, assisting in relaxation and stress reduction. As with most forms of energy work, it can be done in conjunction with other modalities within larger institutions such as hospitals, hospice facilities, and rehabilitation centers as well as practiced on an individual level. In a study published in 2018, meta-analysis validated the analgesic effects of Reiki, revealing that it has a statistically significant impact on patient reports of pain.[8]

This healing energy is available to everyone, within everyone, and is safe to use with any form of medicine. I frequently refer patients to Reiki classes if they have an interest in energy-healing modalities, as they can gain a valuable framework for energetic self-care, or energy hygiene. Energy hygiene is a daily practice of tuning in to and clearing our energy and is just as common as taking a shower or brushing your teeth. As with any energy modality, once a person is attuned to energy via Reiki, he can use it to help others as well as for self-healing. I am specially trained as a Reiki Master in Usui/Holy Fire Reiki, based on William Lee Rand's method. There are many different lineages and styles of Reiki, and teachers and classes are available on every continent if the experience calls to you. For more information, visit www.reiki.org.

Energy-Clearing Symptoms

AS YOU IMPLEMENT CHANGES using energy-healing methods, you might believe that rainbows, butterflies, and unicorns will automatically follow. I don't mean to be the bearer of bad news, but detoxification symptoms, which we've discussed throughout this book, can result from processes other than Lyme disease. Clearing mental, emotional, or energetic trauma can cause symptoms in the body, and if you are not educated about this fact, the symptoms can induce fear, which is counterproductive to the goal of healing. I explained some of my own difficulty with this process at the beginning of the chapter.

When you start to dig deep with energy modalities, you may bring forward energy that needs to be detoxified. This may come as spontaneous emotional release of negative thoughts or old memories, physical sensations from energy stored in the fascia, or a literal release of toxins in the form of diarrhea. When you feel this intensity, it is best to breathe, let go of tension in your body, and act as an observer, watching your release with compassion. A statement that works well for me in these moments is this: "This is the most loving thing that can happen." I will repeat this sentence like a mantra as the uncomfortable sensations move through and out. This release is not about forcing anything to happen; it's about your ability to be with what is uncomfortable, allow yourself to feel emotions, and watch them pass through.

I needed help from others and some practice to learn how to allow the process instead of resisting it out of fear. The body will implement the most efficient way to release stagnant energy through your meridians, your emotional body, and chakra system; but when the analytical left brain kicks in with worries about the process, psychological ailments, and medical diagnoses, it can bring the process to a halt. Understanding this as a natural process of self-healing can help you step into self-care and determine your limits, understanding that you need to pull back if you touch on emotions or memories that are too intense to handle in the moment.

It is wise to have support medically and psychologically to maintain your ground through the process until you feel you have regained more solid emotional and physical health. Eventually, over time, you can find a more peaceful state of mind, and your baseline for what triggers a stress or fear response will change. You can become more in tune with others if you develop *unity consciousness*, the feeling of being connected, supported, and in tune with your own intuition, with access to physical energy and creativity. The more we clear our conscious and unconscious fears, the less room there is for disease to manifest. The idea here is that if you change yourself, you will improve your personal relationships and those with the broader community in ways you may not even be aware of.

In Summary

I have specialized in tick-borne disease for more than a decade, and I've spent years opening up to the challenges of each case, looking for protocols to treat the infection and offering sincere help for my patients. I also learned much from my journey healing from tick-borne disease myself. I have studied and worked with many modalities to find the path of least resistance to recovery.

I love naturopathic medicine because its boundaries are fluid. Many of our standards are identical to those of conventional medical practitioners with regard to medical ethics, licensure, standards of education, and patient privacy. Naturopathic doctors are frequently misunderstood, dismissed as unqualified, or, in my case, demonized for treating tick-borne disease.

The trade-off is that there is a lot of creativity in my profession, and we weave together all forms of medicine, aiming for the patient's highest good. Many practitioners in different fields, some very conservative, are open to integrating energy medicine modalities into their medical practice. I feel that more profound healing is possible when all forms of medicine are integrated, making all modalities available for those who want and respond to them. Energy healing is just another tool that lets us reconnect with our power and enhances our ability to experience peace, reduce pain, improve clarity, and be open to infinite possibilities. This is how we rise above Lyme disease.

REFERENCE CHARTS

The Foundational Naturopathic Treatment Plan

Following are basic elements that form an effective treatment plan for chronic Lyme disease.

- **Probiotic supplement that provides 200–400 billion colony-forming units (CFU); take at lunchtime and before bed.** This supplement needs to be taken at a different time from antibiotics—at least two hours before or after. It can be taken on empty stomach or with food. You may need to take higher or lower dose depending on the reaction of the gastrointestinal tract. The goal is to have regular bowel movements daily and no signs or symptoms of a yeast infection.
  - **Konjac glucomannan:** A natural dietary fiber, this supplement offers protective benefit to the gut with antibiotic use. It is most supportive to *Bifidobacterium* species (beneficial bacteria) against the use of penicillin and tetracycline medications.[1]

- **Herbal antimicrobial formulations.** The best formula for you is based on your individual needs, and may be either a single-herb form or a combination formula. The most commonly used formulas in my practice are Byron White Formulas, Bio-Botanical Research, Beyond Balance, Research Nutritionals, Xymogen, Lyme Core Protocol, Gaia Herbs, Green Dragon Botanicals, Wise Woman Herbals, Nutramedix, and Herb Pharm.

- **Detoxification support formula.** This is to assist the liver and gastrointestinal tract in moving toxins out of the body. It is important to have a combination of herbs to assist in maintaining healthy hepatocytes and improve flow of bile to release toxins. Bitter herbs (dandelion, burdock root, artichoke) and nutrients to enhance glutathione (cysteine, glutamine, and glycine) will typically be a part of the formulation. Detoxification support can also be in the form of a binder such as bentonite clay or activated charcoal, but be careful to take these away from other medications, as they can significantly decrease absorption.

- **Adrenal support.** The type of support the adrenal glands need depends on whether the glands are to be calmed down or enhanced so their function returns to a healthy level. Those that enhance function are most commonly used; these are taken in the morning.

- **Biofilm busting herbals or proteolytic enzymes (serrapeptase, lumbrokinase).** Take on an empty stomach and at least two hours before eating, if possible; it's best to take it daily, even if you must take it with food. Breaking up biofilm allows the antimicrobials and your immune system to more effectively treat your infection.

- **Anti-inflammatory herbal combination.** The main reason we feel symptoms physically is the body's upregulation of pro-inflammatory signals, called *cytokines*. Many natural remedies can reduce the production of cytokines, which benefits the musculoskeletal system, neurological system, and cardiovascular system.
  - **Herbal antifungals:** Herbal antifungals combat the overgrowth of yeasts and other funguses in the body. A dose of two to four capsules per day is typical for the majority of formulas on the market, including gentian violet, caprylic acid, pau d'arco, and berberine.

ANTIFUNGAL NUTRIENTS

NUTRIENTS	DOSING/BENEFITS
Allicin (garlic)	One 200–600 mg capsule two to three times per day (caution with taking blood thinners)
Berberine	One 500 mg capsule two to three times per day
Caprylic acid	1,000–2,000 mg one to three times per day thirty minutes before eating
Curcumin/turmeric	Range is 18–90 percent curcuminoids, dosing is product specific, but look for higher curcuminoid levels
Magnolol (*Magnolia officinalis*)	200–400 mg (can cause drowsiness, used also as a sleep aid and stress-reducing herb); breaks up biofilm created by yeast and ruptures the cell wall of yeast buds[2]
Neem (*Azadirachta indica*)	One 500 mg capsule two to three times per day, with 20 percent active ingredient
Pau d'arco	1,000–4,000 mg two to three times per day, for one week
Saccharomyces boulardii	One 250 mg capsule one to two times per day with antibiotics

COMMON HERBS AND NUTRIENTS USED FOR DETOXIFICATION SUPPORT

HERBS AND NUTRIENTS	DOSING/BENEFITS
Alpha lipoic acid	Dosing recommended at 600 mg three times daily.[3] Helps support liver under oxidative stress due to exposure of heavy metals, alcohol, and other forms of poisoning
Berberine	Reduction of elevated liver enzymes[4]
Burdock root	Hepatic tissue protection with acetaminophen overdose[5]
Fish oil and black cumin seed oil combination	Study showed the combination of black cumin seed oil and fish oil showed great promise as a hepatoregenerative formulation as well as protective to the kidneys.[6]
Globe artichoke (*Cynara scolymus*)	Assists in regeneration of liver cells,[7] enhancing bile flow,[8] anti-hyperglycemic properties[9]
Green tea extract	Hepatoprotective and supports healthy liver enzyme levels in those with nonalcoholic fatty liver disease[10]
Hoxsey-like Formula (Red clover, licorice, burdock, Oregon grape, cascara, buckthorn, poke, queen's root, prickly ash, wild indigo, potassium iodide)	Start at one drop per day and work your way up to maximum of thirty drops per day added to water. Best when used with medical management with your practitioner. This is not meant for long-term use. Advise no more than two to three weeks at a time with two- to three-week breaks.
Licorice root (*Glycyrrhiza glabra*)	Antiviral especially with hepatitis but also herpes type I/II and cytomegalovirus. Also adrenal supportive due to having similarity to chemical compound of adrenal hormone. Has shown ability to regulate liver enzymes in times of hepatic stress. Can be applied topically for viral lesions such as shingles[11]

HERBS AND NUTRIENTS	DOSING/BENEFITS
Milk thistle	Dosing 100–400 mg in divided doses daily with food. Ideally, 80 percent standardized silymarin.[12][13] Antioxidant preventing toxins from entering liver cells[14]
Sho-saiko-to (Combination of bupleurum, pinellia tuber, Scutellaria root, ginseng, jujube, licorice, and ginger)	Two to four capsules per day dosing away from food. Enhances liver regeneration, important remedy for cirrhotic liver, heals medication-related injuries, enhances natural killer cells, prevents malaria and fevers[15]
Swedish Bitters	½–2 teaspoons one to two times per day to stimulate bile release and stimulate proper digestive function
Triphala Rasayana, Emblica officinalis, Terminalia bellirica, Terminalia chebula	Dosing recommended at 500–2,000 mg daily. Detoxifier of the colon, healing for chemical-induced liver impairment[16]
Turmeric (curcumin)	Dosing recommended at 200–600mg three times daily of standardized extract in capsule form.[17][18] Enhances bile flow and supports healthy digestive lining[19][20]
Yarrow (*Achillea millefolium*)	Hepatoprotective, anti-inflammatory

ANTIMICROBIAL HERBS

HERBS	BENEFITS
Andrographis paniculata	Antibacterial, antifungal, liver protective, antiparasitic, anti-inflammatory, immune stimulating. Anti-malarial activity (*Babesia* species).[21] Inhibits quorum sensing[22]
Armoracia rusticana (Horseradish root)	Antibacterial, antifungal, antiparasitic, anti-inflammatory.[23][24] Reduces biofilm. Effective against oral *Candida albicans* (thrush)[25]
Astragalus membranaceus	Antiparasitic, antifungal, anticancer. Synergistic effect when used with atovaquone (Mepron).[26] Inhibits pro-inflammatory cytokines.[27] Anti-biofilm properties when used with *Astragalus angulosus*[28]
Artemisia annua	Antiparasitic, antifungal. Essential oil has antibacterial, anti-inflammatory, and antifungal properties (topically).[29] Artemisinin used globally as anti-malarial medication, enhancing the activation of common pharmaceutical medications such as artemether/lumefantrine (Coartem).
Bacopa (apigenin)	Neuroprotective, anti-inflammatory, antibacterial, antifungal. Contains active ingredient apigenin, shown to enhance the effectiveness of ceftriaxone and ampicillin.[30] Bacoside A, active compound in bacopa, has been shown to have biofilm disruption activity in vitro.[31]
Banderol (Otoba parvifolia) and Cat's claw (*Uncaria tomentosa*)	Antibacterial activity with *Borrelia*, antiprotozoal activity with *Babesia* species. Herbs used in combination have synergistic action with increased ability to kill *Borrelia burgdorferi* by 90 percent and biofilm production.[32]

ANTIMICROBIAL HERBS *(continued)*

HERBS	BENEFITS
Berberine-containing herbs, Goldenseal, Oregon grape root, Coptis chinensis, Barberry root	*Coptis* can work synergistically enhancing antibiotic action, decreasing bacterial adhesion and invasion.[33] *Goldenseal* inhibits efflux pump action in biofilm.[34] *Berberine* compounds are "natural antibiotic."[35] Antiviral and antifungal
Black walnut	A very commonly used, very bitter anti-parasitic. Works topically with fungal skin infections.[36] Enhances tetracycline and erythromycin[37]
Blue flag iris	A remedy historically used for other spirochetal infections such as syphilis and is also a blood purifier, making it helpful with *Bartonella/Babesia* infections
Clove (*Syzygium aromaticum*)	Antibacterial, antifungal, and antiviral activity, analgesic when used topically for tooth pain. Is used both as essential oil and tincture[38]
Grapefruit seed extract	Antimicrobial action with spirochetes, biofilm, and cyst form of *Borrelia burgdorferi*[39]
Houttuynia	Immune modulator, antiviral, antibacterial, and reduced symptoms associated with allergy. Most frequently used with *Bartonella* infection
Japanese knotweed	Antibacterial, anti-inflammatory, anti-hyperlipidemic.[40] Provides a promising antimicrobial agent against drug-resistant bacteria[41]
Lomatium dissectum	Antiviral,[42] expectorant, immune stimulant
Mullein	Anti-inflammatory, antiviral, antifungal, antibacterial, antitumor, expectorant.[43] Disrupts bacterial membranes[44]
Nettles	Anti-inflammatory, antiseptic, detoxifier, vasodilator, and antirheumatic. Decreases biofilm formation when used with antibiotics[45]
Nyctanthes arbor-tristis Linn.	Ayurvedic herb used as an anti-malarial medication most indicated for *Babesia* species[46]
Red root (*Ceanothus*)	Effective with pathogens found in the oral cavity such as *Streptococcus*.[47] Supports lymphatic drainage and healing for the spleen[48]
Skullcap (*Scutellaria baicalensis*)	Anti-influenza remedy (H1N1),[49] antibacterial and antifungal activities[50]
Stephania root	It is able work with dopamine receptors to improve psychomotor dysfunction and mood stabilization.[51] It downregulates the genes that express joint invading proteins.[52] Effective in treating herpes simplex viral types I and II[53]
Teasel (*Dipsacus sylvestris*)	Antimicrobial effects tested to be effective with *Borrelia burgdorferi*. Worked best with spirochete form[54]
Medium-Chain Triglycerides (*Cryptolepis sanguinolenta*, *Sida acuta*)	***Cryptolepis sanguinlenta***: Anti-malarial activity. Aqueous extract found to be effective treating malaria, especially with chloroquine-resistant forms; more rapid fever reduction.[55] Improved liver function and reducing infections of red blood cells[56] ***Sida acuta***: Anti-malarial activity attributed to the active compound cryptolepine.[57] Best for *Babesia* species. Liver protective, reducing changes in tissue with chemical stressors[58]

BIOFILM-INHIBITING HERBS AND NUTRIENTS

HERBS AND NUTRIENTS	DOSING/BENEFITS
Armoracia rusticana (Horseradish root)	Biofilm buster for gram-negative bacteria[59]
Bioflavonoids: coumarin, quercetin, rutin, genistein, rosmarinic acid	Inhibited biofilm formation, inhibited bacterial motility[60] Quercetin dosing: 250–500 mg three to four times per day
Garlic and allicin compounds	Best administered in broth or liquid form for more bacteriostatic impact and destruction of biofilm, whereas the alcohol-based tincture has a more inhibitory action on the formation itself.[61]
Hypericum species	Antimicrobial and disabling biofilm production[62]
Panax ginseng	Can reduce quorum sensing, inhibit biofilm and virulence factors. Dosing amount is important depending on the bacterium being treated, ideally a 0.5 percent aqueous solution.[63 64]
Scutellaria and monolaurin	Synergistic effects in combination at breaking down and increase permeability of biofilms colonies of several pathogens especially *Borrelia garinii* and other *Borrelia* species.[65] Supports mitochondrial function
Stevia	Whole-leaf extract used in culture medium showed antimicrobial effects with *Borrelia* species. Was shown to break down the extracellular polymeric substances, reducing its ability to adhere to substances in vitro[66]

ADRENAL-SUPPORTIVE HERBS AND NUTRIENTS

HERBS AND NUTRIENTS	DOSING/BENEFITS
Ashwagandha (*Withania somnifera*)	Supports proper cortisol release, enhancing energy, helpful in children or those with prolonged illness with improved memory and focus, antianxiety properties equal to that of lorazepam, reduced pain, and enhances mitochondrial function[67]
Cordyceps	500–3,000 mg with food. Active ingredient cordycepin has shown antimicrobial activity, improved libido, cardiovascular support, increased cellular energy, immune modulation.[68] Supports mitochondrial function[69]
Dehydroepiandrosterone (DHEA)	10–50 mg per day. Important to have medically managed with blood levels or salivary hormone levels monitored. This can increase testosterone levels in both men and women to unhealthy levels with excessive dosing. This can improve energy, stamina, libido, and cognition.
Holy basil aka tulsi (*Ocimum sanctum*)	This is the herb that has multiple uses. Adaptogenic herb, assisting the nervous system, detox pathways, anti-inflammation, antimicrobial. Drinking the tea can be seen as a form of "liquid yoga" due to its ability to calm the nerves. It's revered in many cultures as the goddess in which every part of the plant is considered sacred.[70]
Licorice root	Glycyrrhetic acid resembles structure of hormones secreted by the adrenal cortex; accounts for the mineralocorticoid and glucocorticoid effects.[71]
Vitamin B6	Increases progesterone and natural corticosteroids in animal models[72]

NATURAL ANTI-INFLAMMATORIES FOR BRAIN AND BODY

ANTI-INFLAMMATORIES	DOSING/BENEFITS
Bacopa	Antioxidant neuroprotection (via redox and enzyme induction), acetylcholinesterase inhibition and/or choline acetyltransferase activation, β-amyloid reduction, increased cerebral blood flow, and neurotransmitter modulation.[73] Hepatoprotective.[74] 200–600 mg per day in capsules from dried herb. Extract in ethyl alcohol (ETOH) 1:2 ratio 10–30 drops per day. Can start at lower dose and gradually increase
Black cumin seed oil (*Nigella sativa*)	This has many benefits including pain management, antibacterial, antifungal, antiparasitic. It has been shown to work in synergy with alpha lipoic acid, L-carnitine to improve blood sugar levels.[75]
Borage oil/black currant oil	200–400 mg of gamma linolenic acid, which is the anti-inflammatory fatty acid
Boswellia serrata	800–1,800 mg three times per day with or without food
California poppy	Another berberine-rich compound that is neuroprotective, anti-inflammatory, and protects the inner lining of the vascular system[76]
Fish oil	1,000–4,000 mg EPA/DHA combined. Effective alternative to ibuprofen use for anti-inflammation.[77] Can reduce inflammation in the brain with balancing microglial response[78]
5-HTP/L-tryptophan	Improve mood and enhancing serotonin in the brain. Coadministration with creatinine can help improve selective serotonin reuptake inhibitor (SSRI)–resistant depression.[79] When there is disruption of the microbiota or inflammation of the bowel, there is disruption in the balance of serotonin levels in the aspects of the brain dictating mood, metabolism, pain, and cognition. **Do not take if using SSRI medications.**
Forskolin (*Coleus forskohlii*)	180–400 mg with at least 10 percent forskolin, two to four capsules per day. Beneficial for Lyme arthritis[80]
Gamma-aminobutyric acid (GABA)	The supplementation of GABA has been conflicting in the research with the ability to cross the blood-brain barrier, but with concomitant dosing with L-arginine, it did show increased ability to do so. Increasing *Lactobacillus* and *Bifidobacterium* increased GABA through the enteric nervous system, as well as vagus nerve stimulation.[81] Oral dosage: 250–750 mg twice per day
German chamomile	Reduced anxiety, depression and improved insomnia. Improves the communication between brain and the adrenal glands[82]
Gingerroot	Antioxidant, anti-inflammatory, anti-nausea. Helps with detoxification, inhibits pro-inflammatory cytokines[83]
Gotu kola (*Centella asiatica*)	750–1,000 mg per day improves cognition, reduces oxidative stress in the brain, neuroplasticity within the amygdala (area of the brain involved in emotional experience), improves learning and memory.[84]

ANTI-INFLAMMATORIES	DOSING/BENEFITS
Gou teng (*Uncaria rhynchophylla*)	Inhibited neuronal cell death, reduced oxidative damage, and increase glutathione.[85] Reduction of amyloid plaques in the brain related to degeneration seen in Alzheimer's.[86] Reduction of anxiety due to enhanced serotonin levels.[87] Cardiovascular vasodilation effects supporting healthy blood pressure.[88] Attention deficit hyperactivity disorder support.[89] Most readily used in aqueous or ETOH solution with daily 250–1,000 mg/kg dosing
Kava kava (*Piper methysticum*)	Kavalactones, active ingredient, improved depression. Analgesic and anesthetic using non-opioid pathways.[90] It can cause rash but is rare. Can enhance the effects of alprazolam (Xanax). 50–70 mg three times daily
Lavender (*Lavandula angustifolia*)	The essential oil has antibacterial, antifungal, and mood-enhancing qualities. Sleep promoter. Aromatherapy and topical use shown to decrease postpartum depression.[91] Inhalation showed enhancement of function in several areas of the brain in women with magnetic resonance imaging, positron-emission tomography scans, increased alpha and theta waves in the brain promoting calm, thus enhancing cognition. Was shown to improve post-traumatic stress disorder–related symptoms with oral dosing for six weeks of 80 mg.[92] Oral dosing: 80–160 mg per day (proper dilution within supplement intended for oral use; do not take essential oil alone)
Light	Most of us know this, but a reminder never hurts. Increases serotonin levels, so the goal is to get outside more. You need only thirty minutes on sunny day (around 10,000 lux) or more time on cloudy day. Can buy bulbs with different values (3,000–10,000 lux). Timing of treatment is dependent on the strength of light. Also reduction of light with blackout shades in bedrooms and no screen time one to two hours before bed will enhance natural melatonin production from the pineal gland.
Lion's mane (*Hericium erinaceus*)	Protects the brain from neurotoxicity by enhancing mitochondrial function in nerve cells[93]
L-theanine	50–200 mg one to two times per day. Enhances alpha brain waves supporting relaxation.[94] Can reduce stress by reducing sympathetic nervous excitation[95]
Magnolia officinalis and ***Phellodendron amurense***	Dosing magnolol at 5–25 g/kg Improved REM sleep.[96] Anxiety-reducing qualities in menopausal women; active ingredient honokiol and berberine.[97] Improve cognition by modification of the neurotransmitters, useful in treating mild to moderate anxiety. Improved adrenal function, improving mental acuity.[98] Magnolia alone was studied and found to have anti-biofilm properties with common bacteria causing dental caries; active ingredient is magnolol.[99]
Malic acid	1,200–3,000 mg dosing, paired with magnesium for added benefit. For symptoms associated with fibromyalgia and chronic fatigue

ANTI-INFLAMMATORIES	DOSING/BENEFITS
Mapalo (Matapalo [*Phoradendrum crassifolium*])	Dosing recommended at 10–30 drops one to two times per day added to water. The data on this revolve around the plant species, the *Ficus thonningii* tree, which is related to Mapalo showing antimicrobial activity as well as neuroprotective.[100]
Melatonin	1–9 mg before bed. Improves sleep quality, increases sleep time, and decreases time it takes to fall asleep.[101] Improved sleep to decrease oxidation of brain tissue; impaired mitochondrial function and neurodegenerative inflammation[102]
Oat (*Avena sativa*)	Improved attention and focus, task completion.[103] Dosing recommended at 1,600 mg
Panax ginseng	200–400 mg dosing. Neuronal anti-inflammatory, reduces premature death of neurons, improved blood flow to the brain with improved vascular support
Pancreatic enzymes	One to three capsules twice daily. It's hard to be concrete with enzyme doses because of the use of different units of measurement. Away from foods. Reduced inflammation in the digestive tract, as foods are more appropriately broken down, thus reducing systemic inflammation
Phosphatidylcholine	Doses range from 300–4,000 mg. Please speak with health professional to find appropriate dosing for your body. This rebuilds myelin and cellular membranes.
Phosphatidylserine	100 mg three times per day. Required for healthy myelin and cellular membranes[104]
Pyrroloquinoline quinone (PQQ)	Increased blood flow to the brain with prevention of age-related changes in attention and memory.[105] Reduces neurotoxicity and neuroinflamation[106]
Resveratrol (*Polygonum cuspidatum*)	One to two 500 mg capsules daily. Can reduce oxidative damage of the brain in combination with curcumin[107]
Rhodiola rosea	Improves neuronal repair by enhancing stem cells in the hippocampus, decreases anxiety, improved cognition, enhances serotonin and inhibits monoamine oxidase.[108] Dose 100–1,200 mg/day (3 percent rosavin, 1 percent salidroside)
Rosemary (*Rosmarinus officinalis*)	Inhibit neuronal cell death, reduction of heavy metals and reduction of brain inflammation in Alzheimer's.[109] Essential oil is antibacterial, antifungal, activity against drug-resistant gram-positive bacteria, *Candida albicans*.[110] **Tea:** 1–2 g per day steeped in boiling water. **Essential oil:** 0.1–1 ml (6–10 percent concentration) massaged into scalp daily or 5 mg/kg. **Extract:** 2–4 ml (1:1) 45 percent ETOH three times daily.
Saffron (*Crocus sativum*)	Doses showed best outcome above 30 mg/day. Many products commonly having approximately 80–90 mg per capsule. Neuroprotective activity increasing glutathione levels in brain, improving health of myelin sheath.[111] Enhanced mood and decreased anxiety[112]

ANTI-INFLAMMATORIES	DOSING/BENEFITS
SAMe (*S-adenosyl-L-methionine*)	Dosing of 600 mg of enteric-coated tablets twice per day. Anti-inflammatory effects equal to COX-2 inhibitors with pain after one month of administration.[113]
Sarsaparilla (*Smilax*)	Pain reliever, antioxidant,[114] anti-inflammatory
Schisandra berry (*Schisandra chinensis*)	Reduces inflammatory markers stimulating microglial response.[115] Improved cognition[116]
Serrapeptase	One capsule one to three times daily away from food. Enzyme which can cross through the digestive lining to have anti-inflammatory effects reducing pain in the musculoskeletal system as well as biofilm-busting effects
St. John's Wort	Enhances GABA, serotonin levels. Please check with a pharmacist or doctor before taking with other prescription medications due to interactions.
Tianma (*Gastrodia elata Blume*)	Neuroprotective effects by modulating serine, improve neurosynaptic plasticity, decrease abnormal body tremor or seizure-like activity especially when used synergistically with *Uncaria rhynchophylla*.[117][118] 1–1.5 g powdered form
Turmeric/curcumin	400–600mg up to three times per day. Can cross blood-brain barrier to reduce microglial pro-inflammatory pathways[119]
Yarrow (*Achillea millefolium*)	Two to four times per day dosing tincture at 30–40 drops in two to four ounces (60–120 ml) of water. In tincture form, anti-inflammatory action, can inhibit breakdown of extracellular tissue over time,[120] and hepatoprotective.[121] Improves symptoms associated with autoimmune encephalomyelitis in mice study due to decreasing pro-inflammatory cells to cerebrum.[122] As a flower essence, it's used for energy protection from electromagnetic wave sensitivities with electronic devices.
Zhi Zi (*Gardenia jasminoides*)	Reduce waking episodes at night.[123] Essential oil has antidepressant activity. Anti-inflammatory effect.[124] Liver protective[125]

ESSENTIAL OILS WITH ANTIMICROBIAL PROPERTIES

This list summarizes benefits attributed to each oil but does not include all the possible benefits. The oils in **bold italic type** show effective antimicrobial activity against *Borrelia burgdorferi* and biofilm in peer-reviewed research.

ESSENTIAL OILS	BENEFITS
Basil	Pain relief, digestive support, debilitating fatigue
Bergamot	***Fevers, superficial wounds, depression, crisis, and fear***
Chamomile, German	Pain relief, female complaints, indigestion, nerve pain
Chamomile, Roman	Infected skin, sunburns, insect bites, mood imbalance
Cinnamon	***Infections, pain relief, supports the healing of sexual trauma, body image issues***
Clove	***Toothaches, pain relief, digestive support, healthy boundaries, childhood trauma, codependency. Improved cognition***[126]
Eucalyptus globulus	Respiratory support, pain, urinary complaints, helps heal feelings of being undeserving
Frankincense	Coughs, nervous asthma. Scars. Mental fatigue. Reducing overwhelm. Enhances meditation. Father energy
ESSENTIAL OILS	BENEFITS
Geranium	Female hormone imbalance. Leaky gut. Grief and emotional crisis
Lavender	Inflammation. Insomnia. Migraine. Anxiety. Helps one communicate feelings to others
Lemon	Lack of appetite, digestive imbalance. Clarity of thought, elevation of mood, reducing critical thoughts
Lemongrass	Muscle pain, ligaments and tendons. Indigestion. Detoxification. Letting go of limiting beliefs
Magnolia	Abdominal pain. Muscle pain. Difficulty with communication and fears
Melissa	Insomnia, stress, anxiety, nervousness
Myrrh	Fungal skin infections, cough, insect bites. Mother energy and helping one feel safe in the world
Orange	Nervous anxiety. Weakness in legs. Detoxification
Oregano	***Antimicrobial effect with B. burgdorferi, reducing muscle pain. Reduces blocks associated with needing to be right. Unbalanced willpower***
Peppermint	Headaches. Inflammation of the bowels. Respiratory infections. Depression, lack of joy, pessimism
Rosemary	Arthritis complaints. Headaches. Fluid retention. Improved cognition. Revival of vital fire
Sage	Effective for gram-negative and gram-positive bacteria
Tea tree oil	Viral and fungal skin infections. Wound healing
Vetive	Muscle tension. PMS. Overworked. Grounding in crisis. Reveals buried emotions
Yarrow	Antibacterial and antifungal properties in the essential oil compound (topical use only)[127][128]

REFERENCES

CHAPTER 1

1 Daniel E. Sonenshine and Kevin R. Macaluso, "Microbial Invasion vs. Tick Immune Regulation," *Frontiers in Cellular and Infection Microbiology* 7 (2017): 390.

2 Peter J. Krause, Durland Fish, Sukanya Narasimhan, and Alan G. Barbour, "*Borrelia miyamotoi* Infection in Nature and in Humans," *Clinical Microbiology and Infection* 21, no. 7 (2015): 631–39.

3 W. Rueben Kaufman, S. Kaufman, and Peter C. Flynn, "Cuticle Expansion during Feeding in the Tick *Amblyomma hebraeum* (Acari: Ixodidae): The Role of Hydrostatic Pressure," *Journal of Insect Physiology* 88 (2016): 10–14.

4 John F. Anderson, "The Natural History of Ticks," *Medical Clinics of North America* 86, no. 2 (2002): 205–18.

5 Daniel E. Sonenshine and Kevin R. Macaluso, "Microbial Invasion vs. Tick Immune Regulation," *Frontiers in Cellular and Infection Microbiology* 7 (2017): 390.

6 Ivo M.B Francischetti et al., "The Role of Saliva in Tick Feeding," *Frontiers in Bioscience* 14 (2009): 2051–88.

7 Lars Eisen, "Pathogen Transmission in Relation to Duration of Attachment of *Ixodes scapularis* Ticks," *Ticks and Tick-borne Diseases* 9, no. 3 (2018): 535–42.

8 Marc D. Abrams and Michael S. Scheibel, "A Five-Year Record Mast Production and Climate in Contrasting Mixed-Oak-Hickory Forests on the Mashomack Preserve, Long Island, New York, USA," *Natural Areas Journal* 33, no. 1 (2013): 99–104.

9 New Hampshire Fish and Game. "Moose Research: What's in Store for New Hampshire's Moose?" (2018). https://wildlife.state.nh.us/wildlife/moose/study.html.

10 Kirby C. Stafford, III, "Third-Year Evaluation of Host-Targeted Permethrin for the Control of *Ixodes dammini* (Acari: Ixodidae) in Southeastern Connecticut." *Journal of Medical Entomology* 29, no. 4, (1992): 717–20.

CHAPTER 2

1 Katharine S. Walter, Giovanna Carpi, Adalgisa Caccone, and Maria A. Diuk-Wasser, "Genomic Insights into the Ancient Spread of Lyme Disease across North America," *Nature Ecology & Evolution* 1 (2017): 1569–76.

2 Thomas S. Murray and Eugene D. Shapiro, "Lyme Disease," *Clinics in Laboratory Medicine* 30, no. 1 (2010): 311–28.

3 TickReport. "Tick-borne Diseases Passive Surveillance Database," 2018, www.tickreport.com/stats.

4 Kit Tilly, Patricia A. Rosa, and Philip E. Stewart, "Biology of Infection with *Borrelia burgdorferi*," *Infectious Disease Clinics of North America* 22, no. 2 (2008): 217–34.

5 Kit Tilly et al., "*Borrelia burgdorferi* OspC Protein Required Exclusively in a Crucial Early Stage of Mammalian Infection," *Infection and Immunity* 74, no. 6 (2006): 3554–64.

6 Alexia A. Belperron and Linda K. Bockenstedt, "Natural Antibody Affects Survival of the Spirochete *Borrelia burgdorferi* within Feeding Ticks," *Infection and Immunity* 69, no. 10 (2001): 6456–62.

7 William T. Golde et al., "Culture-Confirmed Reinfection of a Person with Different Strains of *Borrelia burgdorferi* Sensu Stricto," *Journal of Clinical Microbiology* 36, no. 4, (1998):1015–19.

8 Tammi L. Johnson et al., "Isolation of the Lyme Disease Spirochete *Borrelia mayonii* from Naturally Infected Rodents in Minnesota," *Journal of Medical Entomology* 54, no. 4 (2017): 1088–92.

9 Centers for Disease Control and Prevention, CDC Newsroom, "New Lyme-Disease-Causing Bacteria Species Discovered: *Borellia mayonii* Closely Related to *B. burgdorferi*," Press Release, February 8, 2016, www.cdc.gov/media/releases/2016/p0208-lyme-disease.html.

10 Centers for Disease Control and Prevention, CDC Newsroom, "New Lyme-Disease-Causing Bacteria Species Discovered: *Borellia mayonii* Closely Related to *B. burgdorferi*," Press Release, February 8, 2016, www.cdc.gov/media/releases/2016/p0208-lyme-disease.html.

11 Daniel López, Hera Vlamakis, and Roberto Kolter, "Biofilms," *Cold Spring Harbor Perspectives in Biology* 2, no. 7 (2010): a000398.

12 Thomas Bjarnsholt, "The Role of Bacterial Biofilms in Chronic Infections," *Journal of Pathology, Microbiology, and Immunology* 121 (2013): 1–58.

13 Arunava Kali et al., "Antibacterial Synergy of Curcumin with Antibiotics against Biofilm Producing Clinical Bacterial Isolates," *Journal of Basic and Clinical Pharmacy* 7, no. 3 (2016): 93–96.

14 Jingjing Sun, Ziqing Deng, and Aixin Yan, "Bacterial Multidrug Efflux Pumps: Mechanisms, Physiology, and Pharmacological Exploitations," *Biochemical and Biophysical Research* 453, no. 2 (2014): 254–67.

15 Eva Sapi et al., "Characterization of Biofilm Formation by *Borrelia burgdorferi In Vitro*," *PLoS ONE* 7. no. 10 (2012): e48277, https://doi.org/10.1371/journal.pone.0048277.

16 Daniel J. Cameron, Lorraine B. Johnson, and Elizabeth L. Maloney, "Evidence Assessments and Guideline Recommendations in Lyme Disease: The Clinical Management of Known Tick Bites, Erythema Migrans Rashes and Persistent Disease," *Expert Review of Anti-infective Therapy* 12, no. 9 (2014): 1103–35.

17 Michael J. Cook, "Lyme Borreliosis: A Review of Data on Transmission Time after Tick Attachment," *International Journal of General Medicine* 8 (2015): 1–8.

18 Gregory Bach, "Recovery of Lyme Spirochetes by PCR in Semen Samples of Previously Diagnosed Lyme Disease Patients," International Scientific Conference on Lyme Disease, April 2001, www.anapsid.org/lyme/bach.html.

19 C.L. Williams et al., "Maternal Lyme Disease and Congenital Malformations: A Cord Blood Serosurvey in Endemic and Control Areas," *Pediatric and Perinatal Epidemiology* 9, no. 3 (1995): 320-30.

20 Malgorzata Bednarska et al., "Vertical Transmission of *Babesia microti* in BALB/c Mice: Preliminary Report," *PLoS ONE* 10, no. 9 (2015): e0137731; Katarzyna Tolkacz et al., "Prevalence, Genetic Identity and Vertical Transmission of *Babesia microti* in Three Naturally Infected Species of Vole, *Microtus* Spp. (Cricetidae)," *Parasites & Vectors* 10 (2017): 66.

21 Kim B. Madsen et al., "Seroprevalence against *Rickettsia* and *Borrelia* Species in Patients with Uveitis: A Prospective Survey," *Journal of Ophthalmology* (2017): 9247465.

22 Geeta Ramesh et al., "The Lyme Disease Spirochete *Borrelia burgdorferi* Induces Inflammation and Apoptosis in Cells from Dorsal Root Ganglia," *Journal of Neuroinflammation* 10, no. 88 (2013): 1–14.

23 Thomas Gregor Issac et al., "Autonomic Dysfunction: A Comparative Study of Patients with Alzheimer's and Frontotemporal Dementia—A Pilot Study," *Journal of Neurosciences in Rural Practice* 8, no. 1 (2017): 84–88.

24 Robert B. Lochhead et al., "MicroRNA Expression Shows Inflammatory Dysregulation and Tumor-Like Proliferative Responses in Joints of Patients with Postinfectious Lyme Arthritis," *Arthritis and Rheumatology* 69, no. 5 (2017): 1100–10.

25 Biju Vasudevan and Manas Chatterjee, "Lyme Borreliosis and Skin," *Indian Journal of Dermatology* 58, no. 3 (2013): 167–74.

26 Kurt E. Müller, "Damage of Collagen and Elastic Fibres by *Borrelia burgdorferi*—Known and New Clinical and Histopathological Aspects," *The Open Neurology Journal* 6 (2012): 179–86.

CHAPTER 3

1 TickReport. "Tick-borne Diseases Passive Surveillance Database," 2018, www.tickreport.com/stats.

2 Udoka Okaro et al., "*Bartonella* Species, an Emerging Cause of Blood-Culture-Negative Endocarditis," *Clinical Microbiology Reviews* 30, no. 3 (2017): 709–46.

3 MicrobeWiki, "*Bartonella henselae*," Microbial Biorealm page on the genus *Bartonella henselae*, last edited 2010, https://microbewiki.kenyon.edu/index.php/Bartonella_henselae.

4 James L. Schaller, Glenn A. Burkland, and P. J. Langhoff, "Do *Bartonella* Infections Cause Agitation, Panic Disorder, and Treatment-Resistant Depression?" *Medscape General Medicine* 9, no. 3 (2007): 54.

5 Ricardo G. Maggi et al., "*Bartonella* Spp. Bacteremia and Rheumatic Symptoms in Patients from Lyme Disease–Endemic Region," *Emerging Infectious Diseases* 18, no. 5 (2012): 783–91.

6 Nahed Ismail, Karen C. Bloch, and Jere W. McBride, "Human Ehrlichiosis and Anaplasmosis," *Clinics in Laboratory Medicine* 30, no. 1 (2010): 261–92.

7 Jennifer H. McQuiton et al., "Inadequacy of IgM Antibody Tests for Diagnosis of Rocky Mountain Spotted Fever," *The American Journal of Tropical Medicine and Hygiene* 91, no. 4 (2014): 767–70.

8 Jessica Snowden and Kari A. Simonsen, "Tick, Rickettsia Rickettsiae (Rocky Mountain Spotted Fever)," StatPearls [Internet], 2017, https://www.ncbi.nlm.nih.gov/books/NBK430881/.

9 Eliane Esteves et al., "Analysis of the Salivary Gland Transcriptome of Unfed and Partially Fed *Amblyomma sculptum* Ticks and Descriptive Proteome of the Saliva," *Frontiers in Cellular and Infection Microbiology* 7 (2017): 476, doi:10.3389/fcimb.2017.00476.

10 Carole Eldin et al., "From Q Fever to *Coxiella burnetii* Infection: A Paradigm Change," *Clinical Microbiology Reviews* 30, no. 1 (2017): 115–90. doi: 10.1128/CMR.00045-16.

11 Carole Eldin et al., "From Q Fever to *Coxiella burnetii* Infection: A Paradigm Change," *Clinical Microbiology Reviews* 30, no. 1 (2017): 115–90. doi: 10.1128/CMR.00045-16.

12 Fabiola Mancini et al., "Prevalance of Tick-Borne Pathogens in an Urban Park in Rome, Italy," *Annals of Agricultural and Environmental Medicine* 21, no. 4 (2014): 723–27.

13 Gilbert J. Kersh, "Antimicrobial Therapies for Q Fever," *Expert Review of Anti-infective Therapy* 11, no. 11 (2013): 1207–14.

14 Ludovic Pilloux et al., "The High Prevalence and Diversity of Chlamydiales DNA within *Ixodes ricinus* Ticks Suggest a Role for Ticks as Reservoirs and Vectors of Chlamydia-Related Bacteria," ed. H. L. Drake, *Applied and Environmental Microbiology* 81, no. 23 (2015): 8177–82.

15 Eugene Escrow et al., "Evidence for Disseminated *Mycoplasma fermentans* in New Jersey Residents with Antecedent Tick Attachment and Subsequent Musculoskeletal Symptoms," *Journal of Clinical Rheumatology* 9, no. 2 (2003): 77–87.

16 A.S. Ramirez et al., "Relationship between Rheumatoid Arthritis and *Mycoplasma pneumoniae*: A Case–Control Study," *Rheumatology* 44, no. 7 (2005): 912–14.

17 Sevgi Yimenicioglu et al., "*Mycoplasma pneumoniae* Infection with Neurologic Complications," *Iranian Journal of Pediatrics* 24, no. 5 (2014): 647–51.

18 H.O. Kangro et al., "A Prospective Study of Viral and Mycoplasma Infections in Chronic Inflammatory Bowel Disease," *Gastroenterology* 98 (1990): 549–53.

19 Wangxue Chen et al., "High Prevalence of *Mycoplasma pneumoniae* in Intestinal Mucosal Biopsies from Patients with Inflammatory Bowel Disease and Controls," *Digestive Diseases and Sciences* 46, no. 11 (2001): 2529–35.

20 C.C. Kuo et al., "*Chlamydia pneumoniae* (TWAR)," *Clinical Microbiology Reviews* 8, no. 4 (1995): 451–61.

21 Andrea S. Varela-Stokes et al., "Microbial Communities in North American Ixodid Ticks of Veterinary and Medical Importance," *Frontiers in Veterinary Science* 4 (2017): 179.

22 Patrick Forterre, "Defining Life: The Virus Viewpoint," *Origins of Life and Evolution of the Biosphere* 40, no. 2 (2010): 151–60.

23 Meghan E. Hermance and Saravanan Thangamani, "Tick Saliva Enhances Powassan Virus Transmission to the Host, Influencing Its Dissemination and the Course of Disease," *Journal of Virology* 89, no. 15 (2015): 7852–60.

24 Syed Soheb Fatmi, Rija Zehra, and David O. Carpenter, "Powassan Virus—A New Reemerging Tick-Borne Disease," *Frontiers in Public Health* 5 (2017): 342; E.R. Campagnolo et al., "Evidence of Powassan/Deer Tick Virus in Adult Blacklegged Ticks (*Ixodes scapularis*) Recovered from Hunter-Harvested White-Tailed Deer (*Odocoileus virginianus*) in Pennsylvania: A Public Health Perspective," *Zoonoses and Public Health* 65, no. 5 (2018): 589–94.

25 Tibor Füzik et al., "Structure of Tick-Borne Encephalitis Virus and Its Neutralization by a Monoclonal Antibody," *Nature Communications* 9 (2018): 436.

26 Dace Zavadska et al., "Recommendations for Tick-Borne Encephalitis Vaccination from the Central European Vaccination Awareness Group (CEVAG)," *Human Vaccines & Immunotherapeutics* 9, no. 2 (2013): 362–74.

27 Wolfgang Hammerschmidt and Bill Sugden, "Replication of Epstein-Barr Viral DNA," *Cold Spring Harbor Perspectives in Biology* 51 (2013): a013029.

28 Kate T. Brizzi and Jennifer L. Lyons, "Peripheral Nervous System Manifestations of Infectious Diseases," ed. Jennifer Lyons, *The Neurohospitalist* 4, no. 4 (2014): 230–40.

29 E. Alari-Pahissa et al., "Low Cytomegalovirus Seroprevalence in Early Multiple Sclerosis: A Case for the 'Hygiene Hypothesis'?" *European Journal of Neurology* 25, no. 7 (2018): 925-33.

30 Richard J. Whitley, "Herpesviruses," in *Medical Microbiology*, 4th ed., ed. Samuel Baron (Galveston: University of Texas Medical Branch at Galveston, 1996), www.ncbi.nlm.nih.gov/books/NBK8157/.

31 Larry J. Strausbaugh et al., "Human Herpesvirus 6," *Clinical Infectious Diseases* 33, no. 6 (2001): 829-33.

32 John B. Harley et al., "Transcription Factors Operate across Disease Loci, with EBNA2 Implicated in Autoimmunity," *Nature Genetics* 50 (2018): 699–707.

33 Kate T. Brizzi and Jennifer L. Lyons, "Peripheral Nervous System Manifestations of Infectious Diseases," ed. Jennifer Lyons, *The Neurohospitalist* 4, no. 4 (2014): 230–40.

34 Jeffrey I. Cohen et al., "Characterization and Treatment of Chronic Active Epstein-Barr Virus Disease: A 28-Year Experience in the United States," *Blood* 117, no. 22 (2011): 5835–49.

35 Jürgen Schulze and Ulrich Sonnenborn, "Yeasts in the Gut: From Commensals to Infectious Agents," *Deutsches Ärzteblatt International* 106, no. 51–52 (2009): 837–42; Franziska Gerwien et al., "The Fungal Pathogen *Candida glabrata* Does Not Depend on Surface Ferric Reductases for Iron Acquisition," *Frontiers in Microbiology* 8 (2017): 1055.

36 Mary J. Homer et al., "Babesiosis," *Clinical Microbiology Reviews* 13, no. 3 (2000): 451–69.

37 Robert E. Quick, "Babesiosis in Washington State: A New Species of Babesia?" *Annals of Internal Medicine* 119, no. 4 (1993): 284–90.

38 FDA News Release, "FDA Approves First Tests to Screen for Tick-Borne Parasite in Whole Blood and Plasma to Protect the U.S. Blood Supply," Press Release, March 6, 2018, www.fda.gov/NewsEvents/Newsroom/PressAnnouncements/ucm599782.htm.

39 I. J. Udeinya et al., "An Antimalarial Extract from Neem Leaves Is Antiretroviral," *Transactions of the Royal Society of Travel Medicine & Hygiene* 98, no. 7 (2004): 435-37.

40 Chhaya S. Godse et al., "Antiparasitic and Disease-Modifying Activity of *Nyctanthes arbor-tristis* Linn. in Malaria: An Exploratory Clinical Study," *Journal of Ayurveda and Integrative Medicine* 7, no. 4 (2016): 238–48.

CHAPTER 4

1 Alexis Lacout et al., "Biofilms Busters to Improve the Detection of *Borrelia* Using PCR," *Medical Hypothesis* 112 (2018): 4–6.

2 Raphael B. Stricker and Edward E. Winger, "Decreased CD57 Lymphocyte Subset in Patients with Chronic Lyme Disease," *Immunology Letters* 76, no. 1 (2001): 43–48.

3 Raphael B. Stricker and Edward E. Winger, "Decreased CD57 Lymphocyte Subset in Patients with Chronic Lyme Disease," *Immunology Letters* 76, no. 1 (2001): 43–48.

4 Uday C. Ghoshal, Ratnakar Shukla, and Ujjala Ghoshal, "Small Intestinal Bacterial Overgrowth and Irritable Bowel Syndrome: A Bridge between Functional Organic Dichotomy," *Gut and Liver* 11, no. 2 (2017): 196–208.

CHAPTER 5

1 John N. Aucott, "Development of a Foundation for a Case Definition of Post-treatment Lyme Disease Syndrome," *International Journal of Infectious Diseases* 17 (2013): e443–e449.

2 Monica E. Embers et al., "Variable Manifestations, Diverse Seroreactivity and Post-treatment Persistence in Non-Human Primates Exposed to *Borrelia burgdorferi* by Tick Feeding," *PLoS ONE* 12, no. 12 (2017): e0189071.

3 Gary P. Wormser et al., "The Clinical Assessment, Treatment, and Prevention of Lyme Disease, Human Granulocytic Anaplasmosis, and Babesiosis: Clinical Practice Guidelines by the Infectious Diseases Society of America," *Clinical Infectious Diseases* 43, no. 9 (2006): 1089–1134.

4 Daniel J. Cameron, Lorraine B. Johnson, and Elizabeth L. Maloney, "Evidence Assessments and Guideline Recommendations in Lyme Disease: The Clinical Management of Known Tick Bites, Erythema Migrans Rashes and Persistent Disease," *Expert Review of Anti-infective Therapy* 12, no. 9 (2014): 1103–35.

CHAPTER 6

1 U.S. Food & Drug Administration, "Label Claims for Conventional Foods and Dietary Supplements," last updated June 19, 2018, www.fda.gov/Food/LabelingNutrition/ucm111447.htm.

2 Lorraine Johnson et al., "Severity of Chronic Lyme Disease Compared to Other Chronic Conditions: A Quality of Life Survey," ed. Claus Wilke, *PeerJ* 2 (2014): e322.

CHAPTER 7

1 Institute of Medicine (U.S.) Food Forum, "Study of the Human Microbiome," *The Human Microbiome, Diet, and Health: Workshop Summary* 2 (2013), www.ncbi.nlm.nih.gov/books/NBK154091/.

2 Institute of Medicine (U.S.) Food Forum, "Study of the Human Microbiome," *The Human Microbiome, Diet, and Health: Workshop Summary* 2 (2013), www.ncbi.nlm.nih.gov/books/NBK154091/.

3 Leo Galland, "The Gut Microbiome and the Brain," *Journal of Medicinal Food* 17, no. 12 (2014): 1261–72.

4 Yu-Heng Mao et al., "Protective Effects of Natural and Partially Degraded Konjac Glucomannan on *Bifidobacteria* against Antibiotic Damage," *Carbohydrate Polymers* 181, no. 1 (2018): 368–75.

5 Francisco Guarner, "Prebiotics in Inflammatory Bowel Diseases," *British Journal of Nutrition* 98, no. S1 (2007): S85–S89.

6 Rima Hatoum, Steve Labrie, and Ismail Fliss, "Antimicrobial and Probiotic Properties of Yeasts: From Fundamental to Novel Applications," *Frontiers in Microbiology* 3 (2012): 421.

7 Jürgen Schulze and Ulrich Sonnenborn, "Yeasts in the Gut: From Commensals to Infectious Agents," *Deutsches Ärzteblatt International* 106, no. 51–52 (2009): 837–42.

8 Joan Hui Juan Lim et al., "Bimodal Influence of Vitamin D in Host Response to Systemic Candida Infection—Vitamin D Does Matter," *The Journal of Infectious Disease* 212, no. 4 (2015): 635–44.

9 Pragati Rawat, Swatantra Agarwal, and Siddhi Tripathi, "Effect of Addition of Antifungal Agents on Physical and Biological Properties of a Tissue Conditioner: An In-Vitro Study," *Advanced Pharmaceutical Bulletin* 7, no. 3 (2017): 485–90.

10 Soheil Moghadamtousi Zorofchian et al., "A Review on Antibacterial, Antiviral, and Antifungal Activity of Curcumin," *BioMed Research International* 2014 (2014), article ID 186864, 12 pages.

11 Nils-Otto Ahnfelt and Hjalmar Fors, "Making Early Modern Medicine: Reproducing Swedish Bitters," *Ambix* 63, no. 2 (2016): 162–83, doi:10.1080/00026980.2016.1212886.

12 Michael K. McMullen, Julie M. Whitehouse, and Anthony Towell, "Bitters: Time for a New Paradigm," *Evidence-Based Complementary and Alternative Medicine* 2015 (2015), article ID 670504, 8 pages.

13 Robin DiPasquale, "Herbs as Bitters: It's a Matter of Degree," January 19, 2009, http://ndnr.com/womens-health/herbs-as-bitters-its-a-matter-of-degree/.

14 Sarah E. Edwards et al., "Dandelion," in *Phytopharmacy: An Evidence-Based Guide to Herbal Medicinal Products* (Chichester, West Sussex [U.K.]: John Wiley & Sons, 2015), 129.

15 Joseph Pizzorno, "Glutathione!" *Integrative Medicine: A Clinician's Journal* 13, no. 1 (2014): 8–12.

16 Ademola C. Famurewa et al., "Dietary Supplementation with Virgin Coconut Oil Improves Lipid Profile and Hepatic Antioxidant Status and Has Potential Benefits on Cardiovascular Risk Indices in Normal Rats," *Journal of Dietary Supplements* 15, no. 3 (2018): 330–42.

17 John W. Newcomer, Nuri B. Farber, and John W. Olney, "NMDA Receptor Function, Memory, and Brain Aging," *Dialogues in Clinical Neuroscience* 2, no. 3 (2000): 219–32.

18 Willmann Liang et al., "Current Evidence of Chinese Herbal Constituents with Effectson NMDA Receptor Blockade," *Pharmaceuticals* 6, no. 8 (2013): 1039–54.

CHAPTER 8

1 Mary Norval, "A Short Circular History of Vitamin D from Its Discovery to Its Effects," *Res Medica* 268, no. 2 (2005): 57–58.

2 Meg Mangin, Rebecca Sinha, and Kelly Fincher, "Inflammation and Vitamin D: The Infection Connection," *Inflammation Research* 63, no. 10 (2014): 803–19.

3 S.P Yenamandra et al., "Expression Profile of Nuclear Receptors upon Epstein-Barr Virus Induced B Cell Transformation," *Experimental Oncology* 31, no. 2 (2009): 92–96.

4 Yongzhong Xu et al., "Using a cDNA Microarray to Study Cellular Gene Expression Altered by *Mycobacterium tuberculosis*," *Chinese Medical Journal* 116, no.7 (2003): 1070–73. et al.,

5 Timothy E. Welty, Adrienne Luebke, and Barry E. Gidal, "Cannabidiol: Promise and Pitfalls," *Epilepsy Currents* 14, no. 5 (2014): 250–52.

6 Garth L. Nicolson, "Mitochondrial Dysfunction and Chronic Disease: Treatment with Natural Supplements," *Integrative Medicine: A Clinician's Journal* 13, no. 4 (2014): 35–43.

7 Kari Johnson et al., "Use of Aromatherapy to Promote a Therapeutic Nurse Environment," *Intensive and Critical Care Nursing* 40 (2017): 18–25.

8 Jie Feng et al., "Selective Essential Oils from Spice or Culinary Herbs Have High Activity against Stationary Phase and Biofilm *Borrelia burgdorferi*," *Frontiers in Medicine* 4 (2017): 169.

CHAPTER 9

1 Kurt E. Müller, "Damage of Collagen and Elastic Fibres by *Borrelia burgdorferi*— Known and New Clinical and Histopathological Aspects," *The Open Neurology Journal* 6 (2012): 179–86.

2 Christopher D'Adamo et al., "Supervised Resistance Exercise for Patients with Persistent Symptoms of Lyme Disease," *Medicine & Science in Sports & Exercise* 47, no. 11 (2015): 2291–98.

3 Roger Jahnke et al., "A Comprehensive Review of Health Benefits of Qigong and Tai Chi," *American Journal of Health Promotion* 24, no. 6 (2010): e1–e25.

4 Ju-Hyun Jeon et al., "A Feasibility Study of Moxibustion for Treating Anorexia and Improving Quality of Life in Patients with Metastatic Cancer: A Randomized Sham-Controlled Trial," *Integrative Cancer Therapies* 16, no. 1 (2017): 118–25.

5 Sven Å Bood, Anette Kjellgren, and Torsten Norlander, "Treating Stress-Related Pain with the Flotation Restricted Environmental Stimulation Technique: Are There Differences between Women and Men?" *Pain Research & Management: The Journal of the Canadian Pain Society* 14, no. 4 (2009): 293–98.

6 C. Michael Dunham, Jesse V. McClain, and Amanda Burger, "Comparison of Bispectral Index™ Values during the Flotation Restricted Environmental Stimulation Technique and Results for Stage I Sleep: A Prospective Pilot Investigation," *BMC Research Notes* 10 (2017): 640.

7 Bruno Bordoni et al., "Emission of Biophotons and Adjustable Sounds by the Fascial System: Review and Reflections for Manual Therapy," *Journal of Evidence-Based Integrative Medicine* 23 (2018): 2515690X17750750.

8 Yuji Soejima et al., "Effects of Waon Therapy on Chronic Fatigue Syndrome: A Pilot Study," *Internal Medicine* 54 (2015): 333–38.

9 Lino Sergio Rocha Conceição et al., "Effect of Waon Therapy in Individuals with Heart Failure: A Systematic Review," *Journal of Cardiac Failure* 24, no. 3 (2018): 204–206.

10 Shanshan Shui et al., "Far-Infrared Therapy for Cardiovascular, Autoimmune, and Other Chronic Health Problems: A Systematic Review," *Experimental Biology and Medicine* 240, no. 10 (2015): 1257–65.

CHAPTER 10

1 Robert C. Bransfield, "Suicide and Lyme and Associated Diseases," *Neuropsychiatric Disease and Treatment* 13 (2017): 1575–87.

2 Myrna M. Weissman et al., "Families at High and Low Risk for Depression: A 3-Generation Study," *Archives of General Psychiatry* 62, no. 1 (2005): 29–36.

3 Rachel Yuhuda et al., "Holocaust Exposure Induced Intergeneration Effects on FKBP5 Methylation," *Biological Psychiatry* 80, no. 5 (2016): 372–80.

4 Carrie Deans and Keith A. Maggert, "What Do You Mean, 'Epigenetic'?" *Genetics* 199, no. 4 (2015): 887–96.

5 Gwenn A. Garden, "Epigenetics and the Modulation of Neuroinflammation," *Neurotherapeutics* 10, no. 4 (2013): 782–88.

6 Robert C. Bransfield, "Aggressiveness, Violence, Homicidality, Homicide, and Lyme Disease," *Neuropsychiatric Disease and Treatment* 14 (2018): 693–713.

7 Emeran A. Mayer, "Gut Feelings: The Emerging Biology of Gut-Brain Communication," *Nature Reviews Neuroscience* 12, no. 8 (2011): 453–66, doi:10.1038/nrn3071.

8 Stephen W. Porges, "Neuroception: A Subconscious System for Detecting Threats and Safety," *Zero to Three (J)* 24, no. 5 (2004): 19–24, http://se-foreningen.no/wp-content/uploads/2016/09/neuroception.pdf.

9 Norman Farb et al., "Interoception, Contemplative Practice, and Health," *Frontiers in Psychology* 6 (2015): 763.

CHAPTER 11

1 Jennifer E. Stellar et al., "Positive Affect and Markers of Inflammation: Discrete Positive Emotions Predict Lower Levels of Inflammatory Cytokines," *Emotion* 15, no. 2 (2015): 129–33.

2 Seth Lloyd, "Quantum Coherence in Biological Systems," *Journal of Physics: Conference Series* 302 (2011): 1–5.

3 Richard Hammerschlag et al., "Biofield Physiology: A Framework for an Emerging Discipline," *Global Advances in Health and Medicine* 4 (2015): 35–41.

4 Fernando Sarmento et al., "Effectiveness of Biofield Therapy for Patients Diagnosed with Fibromyalgia," *Alternative Therapies in Health and Medicine* 23, no. 7 (2017): n.p.

5 Shamini Jain et al., "Clinical Studies of Biofield Therapies: Summary, Methodological Challenges, and Recommendations," *Global Advances in Health and Medicine* 4, Supplement (2015): 58–66.

6 Eugene Rosenburg and Ilana Zilber-Rosenberg, "The Hologenome Concept of Evolution after 10 Years," *Microbiome* 6 (2018): 78.

7 Lynn Margulis, "Symbiogenesis and Symbionticism," in *Symbiosis as a Source of Evolutionary Innovation: Speciation and Morphogenesis*, ed. Lynn Margulis and René Fester (Cambridge: MIT Press, 1991), 1–14.

8 Melike Demir Dogan, "The Effect of Reiki on Pain: A Meta-Analysis," *Complementary Therapies in Clinical Practice* 31 (2018): 384–87.

REFERENCE CHARTS

1 Yu-Heng Mao et al, "Protective Effects of Natural and Partially Degraded Konjac Glucomannan on *Bifidobacteria* against Antibiotic Damage." *Carbohydrate Polymers* 181 (2018): 368–75.

2 Jawad Behbehani et al., "The Natural Compound Magnolol Affects Growth, Biofilm Formation, and Ultrastructure of Oral *Candida* Isolates," *Microbial Pathogenesis* 133 (2017): 209–17.

3 Juanita Bustamante et al., "α-Lipoic Acid in Liver Metabolism and Disease," *Free Radical Biology and Medicine* 24, no. 6 (1998): 1023–39.

4 Xiaoyun Wei et al., "The Therapeutic Effect of Berberine in the Treatment of Nonalcoholic Fatty Liver Disease: A Meta-Analysis," *Evidence-Based Complementary and Alternative Medicine,* 2016 (2016), article ID 3593951, 9 pages.

5 Attalla Farag El-Kott and Mashael Mohammed Bin-Meferij, "Use of *Arctium lappa* Extract against Acetaminophen-Induced Hepatotoxicity in Rats," *Current Therapeutic Research, Clinical and Experimental* 77 (2015): 73–78.

6 Sahar Y. Al-Okbi et al., "Hepatic Regeneration and Reno-Protection by Fish Oil, *Nigella sativa* Oil and Combined Fish Oil/*Nigella sativa* Volatiles in CCl4 Treated Rats," *Journal of Oleo Science* 67, no. 3 (2018): 345–53.

7 Emine Colak et al., "The Hepatocurative Effects of *Cynara scolymus* L. Leaf Extract on Carbon Tetrachloride-Induced Oxidative Stress and Hepatic Injury in Rats," *SpringerPlus* 5 (2016): 216.

8 Maryem Ben Salem et al., "Pharmacological Studies of Artichoke Leaf Extract and Their Health Benefits," *Plant Foods for Human Nutrition* 70 (2015): 441.

9 Maryem Ben Salem et al., "Protective Effects of *Cynara scolymus* Leaves Extract on Metabolic Disorders and Oxidative Stress in Alloxan-Diabetic Rats," *BMC Complementary and Alternative Medicine* 17 (2017): 328.

10 Ali Pezeshki et al., "The Effect of Green Tea Extract Supplementation on Liver Enzymes in Patients with Nonalcoholic Fatty Liver Disease," *International Journal of Preventive Medicine* 7 (2016): 28.

11 A.G. Morgan and W.A. McAdam, "*Glycyrrhiza glabra* Monograph," *Alternative Medicine Review* 10, no. 3 (2005): 230–37.

12 Christopher Hobbs, *Natural Therapy for Your Liver: Herbs and Other Natural Remedies for a Healthy Liver*, 2nd ed. (New York: Avery, 2002), 117.

13 Drugs.com, "Milk Thistle," September 18, 2017, https://www.drugs.com/npp/milk-thistle.html.

14 Ludovico Abenavoli et al., "Milk Thistle in Liver Diseases: Past, Present, Future," *Phytotherapy Research* 24 (2010): 1423–32.

15 Memorial Sloan Kettering Cancer Center, "Sho-saiko-to," February 7, 2014, www.mskcc.org/cancer-care/integrative-medicine/herbs/sho-saiko.

16 Dewasya Pratap Singh and Dayanandan Mani, "Protective Effect of *Triphala Rasayana* against Paracetamol-Induced Hepato–Renal Toxicity in Mice," *Journal of Ayurveda and Integrative Medicine* 6, no. 3 (2015): 181–86.

17 Turmeric for Health, "Ideal Turmeric Dosage: How Much Turmeric Can You Take in a Day," n.d., www.turmericforhealth.com.

18 Subash C. Gupta, Sridevi Patchva, and Bharat B. Aggarwal, "Therapeutic Roles of Curcumin: Lessons Learned from Clinical Trials," *The AAPS Journal* 15, no. 1 (2013): 195–218.

19 Sahdeo Prasad and Bharat B. Aggarwal, "Turmeric, the Golden Spice: From Traditional Medicine to Modern Medicine," in *Herbal Medicine: Biomolecular and Clinical Aspects*, 2nd ed., ed. Iris F.F. Benzie and Sissi Wachtel-Galor (Boca Raton, FL: CRC Press/Taylor & Francis, 2011), 263–88.

20 Yadira Rivera-Espinoza et al., "Pharmacological Actions of Curcumin in Liver Diseases or Damage," *Liver International* 29, no. 10 (2009): 1457–66.

21 Agbonlahor Okhuarobo et al., "Harnessing the Medicinal Properties of *Andrographis paniculata* for Diseases and Beyond: A Review of Its Phytochemistry and Pharmacology," *Asian Pacific Journal of Tropical Disease* 4, no. 3 (2014): 213–22.

22 Malabika Banerjee et al., "Attenuation of *Psuedomonas aeruginosa* Quorum Sensing, Virulence and Biofilm Formation by Extracts of *Andrographis paniculata*," *Microbial Pathogenesis* 113 (2017): 85–93.

23 Stefania Marzocco et al., "Anti-inflammatory Activity of Horseradish (*Armoracia rusticana*) Root Extracts in LPS-Stimulated Macrophages," *Food & Function* 6 (2015): 3778–88.

24 Corinna Herz et al., "Evaluation of an Aqueous Extract from Horseradish Root (*Armoracia rusticana* Radix) against Lipopolysaccharide-Induced Cellular Inflammation Reaction," *Evidence-Based Complementary and Alternative Medicine* 2017 (2017), article ID 1950692, 10 pages.

25 Ho-Won Park, Kyu-Duck Choi, Il-Shik Shin. "Antimicrobial Activity of Isothiocyanates (ITCs) Extracted from Horseradish (*Armoracia rusticana*) Root against Oral Microorganisms," *Biocontrol Science* 18 (2013): 163–68.

26 Nese Sonmez et al., "Effects of Atovaquone and Astragalus Combination on the Treatment and IL-2, IL-12, IFN-γ Levels on Mouse Models of Acute Toxoplasmosis," *Mikrobiyoloji Bulteni* 48, no. 4 (2014): 639–51.

27 Yan Qi et al., "Anti-inflammatory and Immunostimulatory Activities of Astragalosides," *The American Journal of Chinese Medicine* 45, no. 6 (2017): 1157–67.

28 Hussein Kanaan et al., "Screening for Antibacterial and Antibiofilm Activities in *Astragalus angulosus*," *Journal of Intercultural Ethnopharmacology* 6, no. 1 (2017): 50–57.

29 Fabien Juteau et al., "Antibacterial and Antioxidant Activities of *Artemisia annua* Essential Oil," *Fitoterapia* 73, no. 6 (2002): 532–35.

30 K. Akilandeswari and K. Ruckmani, "Synergistic Antibacterial Effect of Apigenin with β-Lactam Antibiotics and Modulation of Bacterial Resistance by a Possible Membrane Effect against Methicillin Resistant *Staphylococcus aureus*," *Cellular and Molecular Biology* 62, no. 14 (2016): 74–82.

31 Debaprasad Parai et al., "Effect of Bacoside A on Growth and Biofilm Formation by *Staphylococcus aureus* and *Pseudomonas aeruginosa*," *Canadian Journal of Microbiology* 63 (2017): 169–78.

32 Akshita Datar et al., "In Vitro Effectiveness of Samento and Banderol Herbal Extracts on the Different Morphological Forms of *Borrelia burgdorferi*," *Townsend Letter: The Examiner of Alternative Medicine*, Lyme Disease Research Group, University of New Haven (July 2010), www.townsendletter.com/July2010/sapi0710.html.

33 Hyeon-Hee Yu et al., "Antimicrobial Activity of Berberine Alone and in Combination with Ampicillin or Oxacillin against Methicillin-Resistant *Staphylococcus aureus*," *Journal of Medicinal Food* 8, no. 4 (2005): 454–61.

34 Kevin A. Ettefagh et al., "Goldenseal (*Hydrastis Canadensis* L.) Extracts Synergistically Enhance the Antibacterial Activity of Berberine via Efflux Pump Inhibition," *Planta Medica* 77, no. 8 (2011): 835–40.

35 Matthew Wood, *The Book of Herbal Wisdom: Using Plants as Medicines*, (Berkeley, CA: North Atlantic Books, 1997), 293–394.

36 Alice M. Clark, Tannis M. Jurgens, and Charles D. Hufford, "Antimicrobial Activity of Juglone," *Phytotherapy Research* 4, no. 1(1990): 11–14.

37 Tarek Zmantar et al., "Use of Juglone as Antibacterial and Potential Efflux Pump Inhibitors in *Staphylococcus aureus* Isolated from the Oral Cavity." *Microbial Pathogenesis* 101 (2016): 44–49.

38 Diego Francisco Cortés-Rojas, Claudia Regina Fernandes de Souza, and Wanderley Pereira Oliveira, "Clove (*Syzygium aromaticum*): A Precious Spice," *Asian Pacific Journal of Tropical Biomedicine* 4, no. 2 (2014): 90–96.

39 Anna Goc and Matthias Rath, "The Anti-Borreliae Efficacy of Phytochemicals and Micronutrients: An Update," *Therapeutic Advances in Infectious Disease* 3, no. 3–4 (2016): 75–82.

40 Wei Peng, Rongxin Qin, Xiaoli Li, and Hong Zhou, "Botany, Phytochemistry, Pharmacology, and Potential Application of *Polygonum cuspidatum* Sieb.et Zucc.: A Review," *Journal of Ethnopharmacology* 148 (2013) 729–45.

41 Pai-Wei Su et al., "Antibacterial Activities and Antibacterial Mechanisms of Polygonum cuspidatum Extracts against Nosocomial Drug-Resistant Pathogens," *Molecules* 20 (2015): 11119–30.

42 A.R. McCutcheon et al., "Antiviral Screening of British Columbian Medicinal Plants," *Journal of Ethnopharmacology* 49 (1995): 101–10.

43 Eibhlín McCarthy and Jim M. O'Mahony, "What's in a Name? Can Mullein Weed Beat TB Where Modern Drugs Are Failing?" *Evidence-Based Complementary and Alternative Medicine* 2011 (2011), article ID 239237, 7 pages.

44 Gorkem Dulger, Tulay Tutenocakli, and Basaran Dulgar, "Antimicrobial Potential of the Leaves of Common Mullein (*Verbascum Thapsus* L., Scrophulariaceae) on Microorganisms Isolated from Urinary Tract Infections," *Journal of Medicinal Plants Studies* 3, no. 2 (2015): 86–89.

45 Zoya Samoilova, "Medicinal Plant Extracts Can Variously Modify Biofilm Formation in *Escherichia coli*," *Antonie van Leeuwenhoek* 105, no. 4 (2014): 709–22.

46 Chhaya S. Godse et al., "Antiparasitic and Disease-Modifying Activity of *Nyctanthes arbor-tristis* Linn. in Malaria: An Exploratory Clinical Study," *Journal of Ayurveda and Integrative Medicine* 7, no. 4 (2016): 238–48.

47 Xing-Cong Li, Linin Cai, and Christine D. Wu, "Antimicrobial Compounds from *Ceanothus americanus* against Oral Pathogens," *Phytochemistry* 46, no. 1 (1997):97–102.

48 Michael Moore, "Ceanothus Red Root," *Southwest School of Botanical Medicine: Medicinal Plant Folio*, n.d., www.swsbm.com/FOLIOS/RedRtFol.pdf.

49 Shuai Ji et al., "Anti-H1N1 Virus, Cytotoxic and Nrf2 Activation Activities of Chemical Constituents from *Scutellaria baicalensis*," *Journal of Ethnopharmacology* 176 (2015): 475–84.

50 Qing Zhao, Xiao-Ya Chen, and Cathie Martin, "*Scutellaria baicalensis*, the Golden Herb from the Garden of Chinese Medicinal Plants," *Science Bulletin* 61, no. 18 (2016): 1391–98.

51 Wei Fu et al., "Dopamine D1 Receptor Agonist and D2 Receptor Antagonist Effects of the Natural Product (?)-Stepholidine: Molecular Modeling and Dynamics Simulations," *Biophysical Journal* 93, no. 5 (2007): 1431–41.

52 L.V. Qi et al., "Tetrandrine Inhibits Migration and Invasion of Rheumatoid Arthritis Fibroblast-Like Synoviocytes through Down-Regulating the Expressions of Rac1, Cdc42, and RhoA GTPases and Activation of the PI3K/Akt and JNK Signaling Pathways," *Chinese Journal of Natural Medicine* 13, no. 11 (2015): 831–41.

53 As'ari Nawawi et al., "Anti-Herpes Simplex Virus Activity of Alkaloids Isolated from *Stephania cepharantha*," *Biological and Pharmaceutical Bulletin* 22, no. 3 (1999): 268–74.

54 Anna Goc and Matthias Rath, "The Anti-Borreliae Efficacy of Phytochemicals and Micronutrients: An Update," *Therapeutic Advances in Infectious Disease* 3, no. 3–4 (2016): 75–82.

55 Michael S. Tempesta, "The Clinical Efficacy of *Cryptolepis sanguinolenta* in the Treatment of Malaria," *Ghana Medical Journal* 44, no. 1 (2010): 1–2.

56 K.A. Bugyei, G.L. Boye, and M.E. Addy, "Clinical Efficacy of a Tea-Bag Formulation of *Cryptolepis sanguinolenta* Root in the Treatment of Acute Uncomplicated Falciparum Malaria," *Ghana Medical Journal* 44, no. 1 (2010): 3–9.

57 Daminoti Karou et al., "Antimalarial Activity of *Sida acuta* Burm. f. (Malvaceae) and *Pterocarpus erinaceus* Poir. (Fabaceae)," *Journal of Ethnopharmacology* 89, no. 2–3 (2003): 291–94.

58 C.D. Sreedevi et al., "Hepatoprotective Studies on *Sida acuta* Burm. f.," *Journal of Ethnopharmacology* 124, no. 2 (2009): 171–75.

59 Stefan J. Kaiser et al., "Natural Isothiocynates Express Antimicrobial Activity against Developing and Mature Biofilms of *Pseudoonas aeruginosa*," *Fitoterapia* 119 (2017): 57–63.

60 Livia Slobodnikova et al., "Antibiofilm Activity of Plant Polyphenols" *Molecules* 21, no. 12 (2016): 1717.

61 Zeinab Mohsenipour and Mehdi Hassanshahian, "The Effects of *Allium sativum* Extracts on Biofilm Formation and Activities of Six Pathogenic Bacteria," *Jundishapur Journal of Microbiology* 8, no. 8 (2015): e18971.

62 S.A. Sarkisian et al., "Inhibition of Bacterial Growth and Biofilm Production by Constituents from *Hypericum* spp.," *Phytotherapy Research* 26, no. 7 (2012): 1012–16.

63 Z. Song et al., "*Panax ginseng* Has Anti-infective Activity against Opportunistic Pathogen *Pseudomonas aeruginosa* by Inhibiting Quorum Sensing, a Bacterial Communication Process Critical for Establishing Infection," *Phytomedicine* 17, no. 13 (2010): 1040–46.

64 Hong Wu et al., "Effects of Ginseng on *Pseudomonas aeruginosa* Motility and Biofilm Formation," *FEMS Immunology & Medical Microbiology* 62, no. 1 (2011): 49–56.

65 Anna Goc, Aleksandra Niedzwiecki, and Matthias Rath. "*In Vitro* Evaluation of Antibacterial Activity of Phytochemicals and Micronutrients against *Borrelia burgdorferi* and *Borrelia garinii*," *Journal of Applied Microbiology* 119, no. 6 (2015): 1561–72.

66 P.A.S. Theophilus et al., "Effectiveness of *Stevia rebaudiana* Whole Leaf Extract against the Various Morphological Forms of *Borrelia burgdorferi in Vitro*," *European Journal of Microbiology & Immunology* 5, no. 4 (2015): 268–80.

67 Narendra Singh et al., "An Overview on Ashwagandha: A Rasayana (Rejuvenator) of Ayurveda," *African Journal of Traditional, Complementary, and Alternative Medicines* 8, no. 5S (2011): 208–13.

68 Hardeep S. Tuli, Sardul S. Sandhu, and A.K. Sharma, "Pharmacological and Therapeutic Potential of *Cordyceps* with Special Reference to Cordycepin," *3 Biotech* 4, no. 1 (2014): 1–12.

69 Xing-Tai Li et al., "Protective Effects on Mitochondria and Anti-aging Activity of Polysaccharides from Cultivated Fruiting Bodies of *Cordyceps militaris*," *The American Journal of Chinese Medicine* 38 (2010): 1093–1106.

70 Marc Maurice Cohen, "Tulsi-*Ocimum sanctum*: A Herb for All Reasons," *Journal of Ayurveda and Integrative Medicine* 5, no. 4 (2014): 251–59.

71 "Monograph: *Glycyrrhiza glabra*," *Alternative Medicine Review* 10, no. 3 (2005): 230–37.

72 Sukanya Jaroenporn et al., "Effects of Pantothenic Acid Supplementation on Adrenal Steroid Secretion from Male Rats," *Biological and Pharmaceutical Bulletin* 31, no. 6 (2008): 1205–8.

73 Sebastian Aguiar and Thomas Borowski, "Neuropharmacological Review of the Nootropic Herb *Bacopa monnieri*," *Rejuvenation Research* 16, no. 4 (2013): 313–26.

74 Sebastian Aguiar and Thomas Borowski, "Neuropharmacological Review of the Nootropic Herb *Bacopa monnieri*," *Rejuvenation Research* 16, no. 4 (2013): 313–26.

75 Aftab Ahmad et al., "A Review on Therapeutic Potential of *Nigella sativa*: A Miracle Herb," *Asian Pacific Journal of Tropical Biomedicine* 3, no. 5 (2013): 337–52.

76 Arrigo F.G. Cicero and Alessandra Baggioni, "Berberine and Its Role in Chronic Disease," in *Anti-inflammatory Nutraceuticals and Chronic Diseases*. Advances in Experimental Medicine and Biology, vol. 928, ed. Subash Chandra Gupta, Sahdeo Prasad, and Bharat B. Aggarwal (Cham, Switzerland: Springer, 2016), 27–45.

77 Joseph Charles Maroon et al."ω-3 Fatty Acids (Fish Oil) as an Anti-inflammatory: An Alternative to Nonsteroidal Anti-inflammatory Drugs for Discogenic Pain," *Surgical Neurology* 65, no. 4 (2006): 326–31.

78 Xiangrong Chen et al., "Omega-3 Polyunsaturated Fatty Acid Attenuates the Inflammatory Response by Modulating Microglia Polarization through SIRT1-Mediated Deacetylation of the HMGB1/NF-κB Pathway Following Experimental Traumatic Brain Injury," *Journal of Neuroinflammation* 15 (2018): 116.

79 Brent M. Kious et al., "An Open-Label Pilot Study of Combined Augmentation with Creatine Monohydrate and 5-Hydroxytryptophan for Selective Serotonin Reuptake Inhibitor– or Serotonin-Norepinephrine Reuptake Inhibitor–Resistant Depression in Adult Women," *Journal of Clinical Psychopharmacology* 37, no. 5 (2017): 578–83.

80 Hua Zhao et al., "Isoforskolin Downregulates Proinflammatory Responses Induced by *Borrelia burgdorferi* Basic Membrane Protein A," *Experimental and Therapeutic Medicine* 14, no.6 (2017): 5974–80.

81 Evert Boonstra et al., "Neurotransmitters as Food Supplements: The Effects of GABA on Brain and Behavior," *Frontiers in Psychology* 6 (2015): 1520.

82 Lei Liu et al., "Herbal Medicine for Anxiety, Depression and Insomnia," *Current Neuropharmacology* 13, no. 4 (2015): 481–93.

83 Ann M. Bode and Zigang Dong. "The Amazing and Mighty Ginger," in *Herbal Medicine: Biomolecular and Clinical Aspects*, 2nd ed., ed. Iris F. F. Benzie and Sissi Wachtel-Galor (Boca Raton, FL: CRC Press/Taylor & Francis, 2011), 131–56.

84 Kun Marisa Farhana et al., "Effectiveness of Gotu Kola Extract 750?mg and 1000?mg Compared with Folic Acid 3?mg in Improving Vascular Cognitive Impairment after Stroke," *Evidence-Based Complementary and Alternative Medicine* 2016 (2016), article ID 2795915, 6 pages.

85 Jin Sup Shim et al., "Effects of the Hook of *Uncaria rhynchophylla* on Neurotoxicity in the 6-Hydroxydopamine Model of Parkinson's Disease," *Journal of Ethnopharmacology* 126, no. 2 (2009): 361–65.

86 Hironori Fujiwara et al., "*Uncaria rhynchophylla*, a Chinese Medicinal Herb, Has Potent Antiaggregation Effects on Alzheimer's β-Amyloid Proteins," *Journal of Neuroscience Research* 84, no. 2 (2006): 427–33.

87 Ji Wook Jung et al., "Anxiolytic Effects of the Aqueous Extract of *Uncaria rhynchophylla*," *Journal of Ethnopharmacology* 108, no. 2 (2006): 193–97.

88 Yean Chun Loh et al., "Mechanism of Action of *Uncaria rhynchophylla* Ethanolic Extract for Its Vasodilatory Effects," *Journal of Medicinal Food* 20, no. 9 (2017): 895–911.

89 Hemant K. Singh, "Brain Enhancing Ingredients from Ayurvedic Medicine: Quintessential Example of *Bacopa monniera*, a Narrative Review," *Nutrients* 5, no. 2 (2013): 478–97.

90 "Monograph: *Piper methysticum* (kava kava)," *Alternative Medicine Review* 3, no. 6 (1998): 458–60.

91 Gihyun Lee and Hyunsu Bae, "Therapeutic Effects of Phytochemicals and Medicinal Herbs on Depression," *BioMed Research International* 2017 (2017), article ID 6596241, 11 pages.

92 Peir Hossein Koulivand, Maryam Khaleghi Ghadiri, and Ali Gorji, "Lavender and the Nervous System," *Evidence-Based Complementary and Alternative Medicine* 2013 (2013), article ID 681304, 10 pages.

93 Junrong Zhang et al., "The Neuroprotective Properties of *Hericium erinaceus* in Glutamate-Damaged Differentiated PC12 Cells and an Alzheimer's Disease Mouse Model," ed. Katalin Prokai-Tatrai, *International Journal of Molecular Sciences* 17, no. 11 (2016): 1810.

94 Anna C. Nobre, Anling Rao, and Gail N. Owen, "L-Theanine, a Natural Constituent in Tea, and Its Effect on Mental State," *Asia Pacific Journal of Clinical Nutrition* 17, suppl. 1 (2008): 167–68.

95 Kenta Kimura et al., "L-Theanine Reduces Psychological and Physiological Stress Responses," *Biological Psychology* 74, no. 1 (2007): 39–45.

96 Chang-Rui Chen et al., "Magnolol, a Major Bioactive Constituent of the Bark of *Magnolia officinalis*, Induces Sleep via the Benzodiazepine Site of GABA(a) Receptor in Mice," *Neuropharmacology* 63, no. 6 (2012): 1191–99.

97 Douglas S. Kalman et al., "Effect of a Proprietary *Magnolia* and *Phellodendron* Extract on Stress Levels in Healthy Women: A Pilot, Double-Blind, Placebo-Controlled Clinical Trial," *Nutrition Journal* 7 (2008): 11.

98 Shawn M. Talbott, Julie A. Talbott, and Mike Pugh, "Effect of *Magnolia officinalis* and *Phellodendron amurense* (Relora®) on Cortisol and Psychological Mood State in Moderately Stressed Subjects," *Journal of the International Society of Sports Nutrition* 10 (2013): 37.

99 Yuuki Sakaue et al., "Anti-biofilm and Bactericidal Effects of Magnolia Bark-Derived Magnolol and Honokiol on *Streptococcus mutans*," *Microbiology and Immunology* 60, no. 1 (2016): 10–16.

100 Rachael Dangarembizi et al., "Phytochemistry, Pharmacology and Ethnomedicinal Uses of *Ficus thonningii* (Blume Moraceae): A Review." *African Journal of Traditional, Complementary, and Alternative Medicines* 10, no. 2 (2013): 203–12.

101 Eduardo Ferracioli-Oda, Ahmad Qawasmi, and Michael H. Bloch, "Meta-Analysis: Melatonin for the Treatment of Primary Sleep Disorders," ed. Andrej A. Romanovsky, *PLoS ONE* 8, no. 5 (2013): e63773.

102 Raquel L. Arribas. "Modulation of Serine/Threonine Phosphatases by Melatonin: Therapeutic Approaches in Neurodegenerative Diseases," *British Journal of Pharamacology* 175, no. 16 (2018): 3220–29.

103 Narelle M. Berry et al., "Acute Effects of an *Avena sativa* Herb Extract on Responses to the Stroop Color-Word Test," *The Journal of Alternative and Complimentary Medicine* 17, no. 7 (2011): 635–37.

104 Michael J. Glade et al., "Phosphatidylserine and the Human Brain," *Nutrition* 31, no. 6 (2015): 781–86.

105 Yuji Itoh et al., "Effect of the Antioxidant Supplement Pyrroloquinoline Quinone Disodium Salt (BioPQQ™) on Cognitive Functions," in *Oxygen Transport to Tissue XXXVII*. Advances in Experimental Medicine and Biology, vol. 876, ed. Clare E. Elwell, Terence S. Leung, and David K. Harison (New York: Springer, 2016), 319–25.

106 Chongfei Yang et al., "Pyrroloquinoline Quinone (PQQ) Inhibits Lipopolysaccharide Induced Inflammation in Part via Downregulated NF-κB and p38/JNK Activation in Microglial and Attenuates Microglia Activation in Lipopolysaccharide Treatment Mice," ed. Karin E. Peterson, *PLoS ONE* 9, no. 10 (2014): e109502.

107 Amita Daverey and Sandeep K. Agrawal, "Pre and Post Treatment with Curcumin and Resveratrol Protects Astrocytes after Oxidative Stress," *Brain Research* 1692 (2018): 45–55.

108 Gihyun Lee and Hyunsu Bae, "Therapeutic Effects of Phytochemicals and Medicinal Herbs on Depression," *BioMed Research International* 2017 (2017), article ID 6596241, 11 pages.

109 Solomon Habtemariam, "The Therapeutic Potential of Rosemary (*Rosmarinus officinalis*) Diterpenes for Alzheimer's Disease," *Evidence-Based Complementary and Alternative Medicine* 2016 (2016), article ID 2680409, 14 pages.

110 Suaib Luqman et al., "Potential of Rosemary Oil to Be Used in Drug-Resistant Infections," *Alternative Therapies in Health and Medicine* 13, no. 5 (2007): 54–59.

111 Takashi Ochiai et al., "Protective Effects of Carotenoids from Saffron on Neuronal Injury in Vitro and in Vivo," *Biochimica et Piophyica Acta (BBA)-General subjects* 1770, no. 4 (2007): 578–84.

112 Graham Kell et al., "affron® a Novel Saffron Extract (*Crocus sativus L.*) Improves Mood in Healthy Adults over 4 Weeks in a Double-Blind, Parallel, Randomized, Placebo-Controlled Clinical Trial," *Complementary Therapies in Medicine* 33 (2017): 58–64.

113 Wadie I. Najm et al., "S-Adenosyl Methionine (SAMe) versus Celecoxib for the Treatment of Osteoarthritis Symptoms: A Double-Blind Cross-Over Trial [ISRCTN36233495]," *BMC Musculoskeletal Disorders* 5 (2004): 6.

114 Beatriz Cristina Konopatzki Hirota et al., "Phytochemical and Antinociceptive, Anti-inflammatory, and Antioxidant Studies of *Smilax larvata* (Smilacaceae)," *Evidence-Based Complementary and Alternative Medicine* 2016 (2016), article ID 9894610, 12 pages.

115 Bingyou Yang et al., "Lignans from *Schisandra chinensis* Rattan Stems Suppresses Primary $A\beta_{1-42}$-Induced Microglia Activation via NF-κB/MAPK Signaling Pathway," *Natural Product Research* 23 (2018): 1–4.

116 Bing-You Yang et al., "Effects of Lignans from *Schisandra chinensis* Rattan Stems against $A\beta_{1-42}$-Induced Memory Impairment in Rats and Neurotoxicity in Primary Neuronal Cells," *Molecules* 23, no. 4 (2018): 870.

117 Arulmani Manavalan et al., "*Gastrodia elata Blume* (Tianma) Mobilizes Neuro-Protective Capacities," *International Journal of Biochemistry and Molecular Biology* 3, no. 2 (2012): 219–41.

118 Ching-Liang Hsieh et al., "Anticonvulsive and Free Radical Scavenging Actions of Two Herbs, *Uncaria rhynchophylla* (Miq) Jack and *Gastrodia elata* Bl., in Kainic Acid–Treated Rats." *Life Sciences* 65, no. 20 (1999): 2071–82.

119 Vincenzo Sorrenti et al., "Curcumin Prevents Acute Neuroinflammation and Long-Term Memory Impairment Induced by Systemic Lipopolysaccharide in Mice," *Frontiers in Pharmacology* 9 (2018): 183.

120 Birgit Benedek, Brigitte Kopp, and Matthias F. Melzig, "*Achillea millefolium* L. s.l.—Is the Anti-inflammatory Activity Mediated by Protease Inhibition," *Journal of Ethnopharmacology* 113, no. 2 (2007): 312–17.

121 Muhammad Akram, "Minireview on *Achillea millefolium* Linn," *The Journal of Membrane Biology* 246, no. 9 (2013): 661–63.

122 Reza Vaziriejad et al., "Effect of Aqueous Extract of *Achillea millefolium* on the Development of Experimental Autoimmune Encephalomyelitis in C57BL/6 Mice," *Indian Journal of Pharmacology* 46, no. 3 (2014): 303–308.

123 H. Kuratsune et al., "Effect of Crocetin from *Gardenia jasminoides* Ellis on Sleep: A Pilot Study," *Phytomedicine* 17, no. 11 (2010): 840–43.

124 Wenping Xiao et al., "Chemistry and Bioactivity of *Gardenia jasminoides*," *Journal of Food and Drug Analysis* 25, no. 1(2017): 43–61.

125 Kee C. Huang, *The Pharmacology of Chinese Herbs*, 2nd ed. (Boca Raton, FL: CRC Press, 1999), 257.

126 Manoj K. Dalai et al., "Anti-cholinesterase Activity of the Standardized Extract of *Syzygium aromaticum* L.," *Pharmacognosy Magazine* 10, no. 2 (2014): S276–S282.

127 Ferde Candan et al."Antioxidant and Antimicrobial Activity of the Essential Oil and Methanol Extracts of *Achillea millefolium* subsp. *millefolium* Afan. (Asteraceae)." *Journal of Ethnopharmacology* 87, no. 2–3 (2003): 215–20.

128 Chaker El-Kalamouni et al., "Antioxidant and Antimicrobial Activities of the Essential Oil of *Achillea millefolium* L. Grown in France," ed. Eleni Skaltsa. *Medicines* 4, no. 2 (2017): 30.

Acknowledgments

This book was written with every spare hour or few minutes that were available on a daily basis. It was written on planes, during halftime at my children's soccer games, between patients at my clinic, late nights, early mornings, and in the middle of dinner running to my computer to get the words out before they disappeared. Thank you to Steven Greenspan, my children, and my father, William Geil, for your support in accomplishing my goal of experiencing the joy of manifesting a book.

I have such gratitude for the opportunity to work with The Quarto Group. Special thanks to Amanda Waddell, Susan Lauzau, and David Umla for your guidance through the process.

This book is also dedicated to every patient I have had the privilege to work with, even if for a short while. Each and every encounter has been a learning experience improving my practice of medicine. I have learned more from my patients than I ever could from a book or lecture. I hope this book serves as a piece of information to help you on your path of reclaiming your optimal health.

This book came about after being asked to participate as a guest lecturer with a local chapter of the Holistic Mom's Network. Thank you, Esther Roy, N.D., for the invitation to be a speaker. I also have such gratitude for our time working together and how well you managed my clinic when I was on maternity leave with my second child.

My deepest gratitude to Destiny Green, N.D., who completed her year-long residency in my clinic throughout the process of writing this book. She contributed to research and data collection, which was invaluable. I look forward to our continued collaboration in the daily workings of the clinic and excited to watch you evolve as a doctor in the coming years. It's a privilege to be a part of your professional development.

Thank you to my friend and colleague Laura Chan, N.D., L.Ac., for your support over the years. Your friendship and helpful feedback on the manuscript over the course of the year were important for my morale when I needed another set of eyes.

Thank you to my office staff, Michelle Darrow, Becky Stapleton, Kimmie King, and Susan O'Leary. You have all supported me professionally and personally for many years. This book was possible because of your friendship, loyalty, and sisterhood. Thank you for making sure my needs were met through the process and for having infinite patience with me as your boss. Each of you holds such an important role in the inner workings of my medical practice, which allows me to live my dream of being a doctor more fully than I could have imagined.

To my best friend, Arlene Hayes, for your unconditional friendship, honesty, love, and emotional support, and for our daily drive conversations.

To Theresa Anderson, you have my deep gratitude for our friendship, your support, for watching my kids when I need to make time to write, and for your lightness of being in times I was overwhelmed.

To Joan Ruggiero, you hold a special place in my heart. Words are not enough to convey my gratitude for your presence as a teacher in my life, your light, your authentic style, and your devotion to the work is what I strive to emulate. Thank you.

To Ann Acheson, deepest gratitude for your wisdom, moral support, profound healing abilities, how you carry yourself with such grace, and authenticity. You are an amazing teacher in my life and I'm blessed to have your friendship.

I'm a better doctor and person for having these individual teachers in my life to help me learn to blend science and spirit: Georgette Star; Sandra Ingerman, M.A.; Leontine Hartzell; Dick Thom, D.D.S., N.D.; Guan-Cheng Sun, Ph.D.; Gene Ang, Ph.D.; Miguel Ojeda-Rios, M.D.; Esther Mora, D.D., D.MT.; Heather Zwickey, Ph.D.; Naomi Lewis, India Rose Waters, M.A.; Deborah Willimott, and many more, as well as the teachers to come.

Special thanks to trailblazers in tick-borne disease who have helped me in so many ways in the evolution of my medical specialty, Richard Horowitz, M.D., Charles Ray Jones, M.D., Joseph Burrascano, M.D.; Nevena Zubcevik, D.O.; Dietrich Klinghardt, M.D., Ph. D.; Ritchie Shoemaker, M.D.; Robert Bransfield, M.D.; Carrie Chojnowski, N.D.; and Leon Hecht, N.D. As well as many more. Thank you to the International Lyme and Associated Diseases Society (ILADS) for creating community to share ideas, clinical pearls, research, and improve the quality of care for those suffering with tick-borne disease.

Other teachers whom have made an impact on my life through the written word or online learning are Stanislav Grof, M.D.; Robert Gilbert, Ph.D.; Thomas Hübl, Alton Kamadon, J.J Hurak, Ph.D.; Rudolph Steiner, Paramahansa Yogananda, and Swami Muktananda...as well as many more. My heart is so full.

About the Author

Julia Greenspan, N.D., runs the private medical practice Greenhouse Naturopathic Medicine (www.greenhousemedicine.com) and has been treating patients for tick-borne disease in New Hampshire—one of the epicenters for Lyme disease—for more than 10 years. She is a member of the International Lyme and Associated Disease Society (ILADS), the New Hampshire Association of Naturopathic Doctors, and the American Association of Naturopathic Physicians. She has been interviewed as an expert in Lyme disease on both radio and television and has been published in the Naturopathic Doctor News and Review, the national publication for Naturopathic Physicians.

Dr. Greenspan has a background in psychology and social work specializing in crisis management, and uses a personalized, multi-faceted approach in the treatment of Lyme and other diseases. She holds a Bachelor of Science in Psychology from Portland State University in Oregon and is a graduate from the National College of Natural Medicine. She is a patient advocate, Lyme disease survivor, mother of two, energy healer, lecturer, beekeeper, lifelong student, and dark chocolate addict.

INDEX